The New MRCPsych Paper II Practice MCQs and EMIs

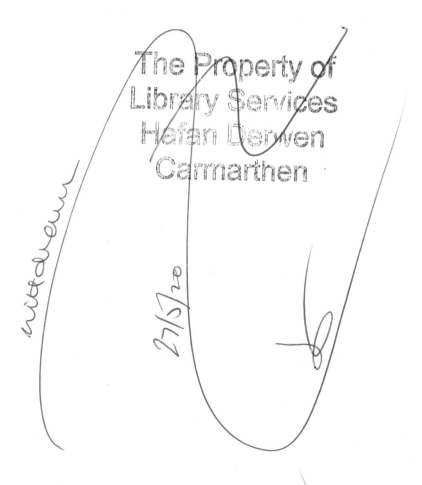

The Property of
Library Services
Hafan Derwen
Carmarthen

The New MRCPsych Paper II Practice MCQs and EMIs

CLARE OAKLEY

MB ChB, MRCPsych

Vice Chair, Psychiatric Trainees' Committee,
Royal College of Psychiatrists
Specialty Registrar in Forensic Psychiatry,
West Midlands Deanery

and

OLIVER WHITE

BMedSci, BM BS, MRCPsych

Chair, Psychiatric Trainees' Committee,
Royal College of Psychiatrists
Specialist Registrar in Child and Adolescent and Forensic
Psychiatry, Oxford Deanery

Radcliffe Publishing
Oxford • New York

Radcliffe Publishing Ltd
18 Marcham Road
Abingdon
Oxon OX14 1AA
United Kingdom

www.radcliffe-oxford.com
Electronic catalogue and worldwide online ordering facility.

British Library Cataloguing in Publication Data

A catalogue record for this book is available from the British Library.

ISBN-13: 978 184619 285 2

Typeset by Pindar NZ, Auckland, New Zealand
Printed and bound by TJI Digital, Padstow, Cornwall, UK

Contents

About the authors

Clare Oakley graduated from the University of Birmingham in 2003 and undertook her basic psychiatric training in Birmingham. She is currently a Specialty Registrar in Forensic Psychiatry in the West Midlands Deanery. Clare has been a member of the Psychiatric Trainees' Committee of the Royal College of Psychiatrists for the last two years and is currently its Vice Chair. She is involved in developing the curriculum and workplace-based assessments within the Royal College of Psychiatrists and so has an extensive knowledge of the assessment system, including the new MRCPsych exams.

Oliver White graduated in 2001 and worked in Nottingham and Sydney, Australia prior to completing his basic psychiatric training on the Mid Trent rotation. He is currently an SpR dual training in Child and Adolescent, and Forensic Psychiatry in the Oxford Deanery. Oliver developed an interest in training issues as an SHO and for the past three years has been a member of the Psychiatric Trainees' Committee of the Royal College of Psychiatrists and is currently Chair of the Committee. He is therefore experienced in the recent changes in psychiatric training, including the development of the new MRCPsych exams.

Introduction

Background

The structure of the MRCPsych examination has changed significantly. The exam will no longer consist of two distinct 'Parts' but will consist of three written papers and one clinical exam. This chapter outlines these changes, and further details can be found on the website of the Royal College of Psychiatrists (www.rcpsych.ac.uk). We recommend that candidates check the website carefully before applying to sit the examinations. This book provides 250 practice MCQs and 100 practice EMIs for paper II.

Examination format

The new written papers will contain 200 questions and will all be three hours long. The papers will include both 'single best answer 1 from 5' style MCQs, and EMIs. The proportion of each type of question in the exam paper may vary but approximately one-third of the questions will be EMIs.

There will be a new OSCE-type examination called Clinical Assessment of Skills and Competencies (CASC). It will consist of two parts to be completed in one day. One circuit will consist of eight individual stations of seven minutes with a preceding one minute of 'preparation' time. The other circuit will consist of four pairs of linked stations, with each station lasting ten minutes with two minutes of preparation time.

Examination content

The topics tested in each paper are shown in the table below. Broadly speaking, paper I can be considered to be similar to the old style Part 1 written paper; paper II has elements similar to the Part 2 basic sciences paper; paper III is similar to the Part 2 clinical sciences paper with additional critical appraisal and statistics.

Paper I	Paper II	Paper III
History and mental state examination	General principles of psychopharmacology (pharmacokinetics, pharmacodynamics)	Research methods
Cognitive assessment		Evidence-based practice
Neurological examination	Psychotropic drugs	Statistics
Assessment	Adverse reactions	Critical appraisal
Aetiology	Evaluation of treatments	Clinical topics
Diagnosis		General Adult
Classification	Neurosciences (physiology, endocrinology, chemistry, anatomy, pathology)	Liaison
Basic psychological treatments		Forensic
		Addiction
Human psychological development	Advanced psychological processes and treatments	Child and adolescent
Descriptive psychopathology		Psychotherapy
Dynamic psychopathology		Learning disability
		Rehabilitation
Prevention of psychiatric disorder		Old age psychiatry
History of psychiatry		
Basic ethics and philosophy of psychiatry		
Stigma and culture		

The proportion of questions in each topic in the chapters of this book is based on the indicative breakdown of questions provided by the College.

Techniques for answering questions

MCQs

- Read the question carefully.
- Watch out for double negatives.
- Narrow down the five options by first excluding those that you know are incorrect.
- Phrases which include 'can' 'may' and 'is possible' are often true.
- Phrases which include 'always' 'never' and 'essential' are often false.
- Understand what the following terms mean:
  - Characteristic: you would doubt the diagnosis without this
  - Typical: same as characteristic
  - Pathognomonic: occurs in that disease and no other
  - Specific: same as pathognomonic
  - Recognised: this has been reported
  - Commonly: more than 50%
  - Rare: less than 5%
  - Almost never: 1–2%

EMIs

Each option may be used once, more than once, or not at all.

Each question may have more than one answer (this will be indicated).

It may be helpful to read the question first before reading the answer options.

EMIs take longer than MCQs to answer – make sure you allow enough time.

Recommended reading

Candidates will have their own preferences about textbooks and revision material. We found the following books useful in our preparation for the Membership exams and they cover most of the material required. In the explanatory notes that accompany the answers in this book, there are references to the books below to enable you to read more fully if you have not understood a topic.

General

Fear C. *Essential Revision Notes in Psychiatry for MRCPsych*. Knutsford: PasTest; 2004.

Gelder MG, Lopez-Ibor JJ, Andreason N, editors. *New Oxford Textbook of Psychiatry (2 Volume Set)*. Oxford: Oxford University Press; 2003.

Johnstone E, Cunningham-Owens DG, Lawrie SM *et al.*, editors. *Companion to Psychiatric Studies*. 7th ed. London: Churchill Livingstone; 2004.

Lawrie SM, McIntosh AM, Rao S. *Critical Appraisal for Psychiatry*. Edinburgh: Elsevier Churchill Livingstone; 2000.

Leung WC, Passmore K. *Essential Notes in Basic Sciences for the MRCPsych Part 2*. Oxford: Radcliffe Publishing; 2004.

Levi MI. *Basic Notes in Psychiatry*. 4th ed. Oxford: Radcliffe Publishing; 2005.

Puri BK, Hall AD. *Revision Notes in Psychiatry*. 2nd revised ed. London: Hodder Arnold; 2004.

Psychology

Gross R. *Psychology: the science of mind and behaviour*. 4th revised ed. London: Hodder Arnold; 2001.

Gupta D, Gupta RM, editors. *Psychology for Psychiatrists*. Chichester: John Wiley & Sons; 1999.

Psychopharmacology

Anderson IM, Reid IC, editors. *Fundamentals of Clinical Psychopharmacology*. 3rd revised ed. Abingdon: Taylor & Francis; 2006.

Levi MI. *Basic Notes in Psychopharmacology*. 4th ed. Oxford: Radcliffe Publishing; 2007.

Taylor D, Paton C, Kerwin R. *The Maudsley 2005–2006 Prescribing Guidelines*. Abingdon: Taylor & Francis; 2005.

Advanced psychopharmacology and therapeutics

Questions

MCQs

1 Which of the following antiepileptics is not a recognised mood stabiliser?

   a Carbamazepine

   b Sodium valproate

   c Lamotrigine

   d Vigabatrin

   e Topiramate

2 Which of the following benzodiazepines is short acting (< 24 hours)?

   a Diazepam

   b Alprazolam

   c Temazepam

   d Oxazepam

   e Nitrazepam

3 Which of the following are not pharmacokinetic interactions between drugs?

a Enzyme induction

b Synergism

c Enzyme inhibition

d Displacement from binding sites

e Chelation

4 Which of the following would you not expect a patient to report as a side effect of tricyclic antidepressants?

a Tremor

b Weight loss

c Black tongue

d Abnormal liver function tests

e Blood sugar changes

5 Which of the following is not indicated for treatment of depression?

a Fluoxetine

b Mirtazapine

c Reboxetine

d Duloxetine

e Zotepine

6 Which of the following half-lives is correct?

a Citalopram – 20 hours

b Fluvoxamine – 200 hours

c Paroxetine – 20 hours

d Sertraline – 12 hours

e Escitalopram – 48 hours

7 Which of the following are not pharmacodynamic interactions between drugs?

a Inhibition of drug uptake

b Interaction at receptors

   c Changes in fluid and electrolyte balance

   d Inhibition of drug transport

   e Changes in gastrointestinal tract pH

8 Which of the following is not correct regarding classification of antipsychotics?

   a Trifluoperazine – phenothiazine

   b Chlorpromazine – thioxanthine

   c Risperidone – benzisoxazole

   d Amisulpiride – substituted benzamide

   e Clozapine – dibenzodiazepine

9 Which of the following combinations of drugs and mechanisms of actions are incorrect?

   a Cocaine: inhibits noradrenaline (NA) reuptake.

   b Cocaine: inhibits dopamine (DA) reuptake.

   c Amphetamine: decreases noradrenaline (NA) release.

   d Amphetamine: increases dopamine (DA) release.

   e Benztropine: inhibits dopamine (DA) reuptake.

10 Regarding zopiclone, which of the following is true?

   a It is a diazolobenzodiadepine.

   b It binds to GABA receptors.

   c It is not secreted in breast milk.

   d It is effective in complex partial seizures.

   e It does not suppress REM sleep.

11 Which of the following is not due to blockage of alpha 1-adrenoreceptors?

   a Drowsiness

   b Sexual dysfunction

   c Cognitive impairment

   d Postural hypotension

   e Weight gain

12 Which of the following SSRIs have active metabolites?

a Citalopram

b Fluvoxamine

c Paroxetine

d Fluoxetine

e Escitalopram

13 A patient questions you about the difference between typical and atypical antipsychotics. Which of the following is a typical antipsychotic?

a Clozapine

b Risperidone

c Olanzapine

d Amisulpiride

e Pimozide

14 A patient's relative comes to see you having read about tardive dyskinesia on the internet. Which of the following is false regarding tardive dyskinesia?

a It is more common in elderly females.

b It can be caused by stopping antipsychotics.

c It was not described before the advent of psychotropic medication.

d It is more common in patients with affective disorder than schizophrenia.

e Clozapine is a potent cause.

15 Which of the following transmitters and precursors are not correctly paired?

a Dopamine and tyrosine

b Noradrenaline and adrenaline

c Adrenaline and dopamine

d Glutamate and glutamine

e Serotonin and histidine

16 Which of the following is not a common adverse effect of clozapine?

a Diarrhoea

b Sedation

c Fever

d Seizures

e Hypertension

17 What is the level of evidence for the use of fish oils in schizophrenia?

a Case reports

b Expert opinion

c Open label trials

d Double-blind randomised control trials

e Non-blinded randomised control trials

18 Which of the following has the strongest evidence base for use as clozapine augmentation?

a Sulpiride

b Haloperidol

c Aripiprazole

d Omega-3 triglycerides

e Olanzapine

19 Which of the following classifications is correct?

a Clozapine is an imidazolidinone.

b Amisulpiride is a benzixasole.

c Olanzapine is a thienobenzodiazepine.

d Aripiprazole is a substituted benzamide.

e Risperidone is a quinolinone.

20 A patient asks you about the foods they cannot eat while taking MAOIs. Which of the following foods is safe to eat when taking an MAOI?

　a　Cheddar cheese

　b　Sherry

　c　Avocado

　d　Caviar

　e　Broccoli

21 Regarding lithium, which of the following is true?

　a　It inhibits extracellular phosphatase.

　b　It is indicated in refractory anxiety states.

　c　It increases adenylate cyclase activity.

　d　Its levels are increased by carbonic anhydrase.

　e　It shows great variation in bioavailability with different preparations.

22 Which of the following adverse effects is recognised when the drugs are taken with disulfiram?

　a　Antidepressants: decreased plasma concentration

　b　Phenytoin: psychosis

　c　Metronidazole: increased toxicity

　d　Benzodiazepine: decreased sedation

　e　Anticoagulants: increased bleeding tendencies

23 A GP phones you concerned about the polypharmacy of one of your patients. Which of the following does not reduce the plasma level of antipsychotics?

　a　St John's wort

　b　Carbamazepine

　c　Smoking

　d　SSRIs

　e　Alcohol

24 Which of the following is false?

    a Most psychotropic drugs are lipophilic and are highly plasma protein bound.

    b Highly lipid-soluble drugs pass through the blood brain barrier.

    c The liver metabolises water-soluble drugs to lipid-soluble.

    d Alcohol follows zero-order kinetics.

    e In first-order kinetics the rate of drug elimination is proportional to its plasma concentration.

25 Which of the following is false regarding anticonvulsants?

    a Lamotrigine reduces glutamate levels.

    b Carbamazepine can cause agranulocytosis.

    c Rash is a side effect of lamotrigine.

    d Valproate blocks sodium channels.

    e Valproate can cause alopecia.

26 One of the nurses is concerned that a patient on the ward is showing signs of lithium toxicity. Which of the following is not a sign of lithium toxicity?

    a Fine tremor

    b Convulsions

    c Vomiting

    d Blurred vision

    e Ataxia

27 Which of the following statements about tricyclic antidepressants is true?

    a They prolong the PR interval.

    b They may increase the action of warfarin.

    c They can cause sinus bradycardia.

    d They inhibit the reuptake of 5HT in the postsynaptic neurones.

    e TCAs and MAOIs have a significant pharmacodynamic interaction.

28 Which of the following statements about clozapine is false?

  a It has a selective action on 5HT 1A receptors.

  b It is a more potent D1 receptor blocker compared to other antipsychotics.

  c It is a more potent 5HT2 receptor blocker compared to other antipsychotics.

  d At therapeutic doses haloperidol is a more potent D2 blocker than clozapine.

  e It is a more potent D4 receptor blocker compared to other antipsychotics.

29 You are going to commence a patient on clozapine and are explaining the initial monitoring to them. They ask you for how long they will need to have their blood pressure taken frequently. Which of the following is the correct response?

  a 6 hours

  b 24 hours

  c 1 week

  d 4 weeks

  e 3 months

30 An overweight patient develops schizophrenia and is worried about further weight gain with antipsychotics. Which of the following antipsychotics has the least potential to cause weight gain?

  a Clozapine

  b Chlorpromazine

  c Aripiprazole

  d Olanzapine

  e Risperidone

31 You are called to the ward to assess somebody who the nurses suspect may have neuroleptic malignant syndrome. Which of the following is not a risk factor for this?

a High-potency typical antipsychotics

b Rapid dose increase

c Rapid dose decrease

d Organic brain disease

e Chronic antipsychotic prescription

32 An elderly patient with their first episode of depression also suffers from heart disease. Which would be the safest antidepressant to prescribe?

a Venlafaxine

b Sertraline

c Mirtazapine

d Trazadone

e Amitriptyline

33 A patient you wish to commence on clozapine is reluctant to have regular blood tests. How long are weekly blood tests necessary?

a 4 weeks

b 10 weeks

c 14 weeks

d 18 weeks

e 24 weeks

34 Which of the following statements about benzodiazepines is false?

a They inhibit CP450 enzymes.

b They potentiate the action of GABA.

c They can impair new learning.

d They suppress REM sleep.

e They act via specific benzodiazepine receptors in the brain.

35 A routine lithium level is elevated and you think that the prescription of an additional medication may be the explanation. Which of the following could be the cause?

a Carbamazepine

b Metoclopramide

c NSAIDs

d Haloperidol

e Metronidazole

36 Which of the following decreases plasma levels of clozapine?

a Increased age

b Taking phenytoin

c Being female

d Drinking coffee

e Taking fluoxetine

37 Which of the following statements about tardive dyskinesia is true?

a It is more common in elderly men compared to elderly women.

b It is associated with long-term use of clozapine.

c It is treated with anticholinergics.

d There is an increased risk in patients with bipolar affective disorder treated with antipsychotics.

e It is resolved by stopping the antipsychotic.

38 Which of the following increases the neurotoxicity of lithium without increasing plasma levels?

a ACE inhibitors

b NSAIDs

c Loop diuretics

d Metoclopramide

e Potassium-sparing diuretics

39 Which of the following statements about SSRIs is false?
   a They are more efficacious than TCAs in treating depression.
   b They can cause EPSEs at therapeutic doses.
   c Citalopram is the most selective.
   d They increase sleep latency.
   e They inhibit the CP450 enzyme systems.

40 Which of the following statements about MAOIs is false?
   a They can cause hypertension.
   b They can cause arthritis.
   c Moclobemide is safe in epilepsy.
   d They cause suppression of REM sleep.
   e Cheese can be eaten two weeks after discontinuing them.

41 Which of the following does not occur with chronic lithium therapy?
   a Hypothyroidism
   b Metallic taste
   c Weight gain
   d Renal damage
   e ECG changes

42 Which of the following is false in relation to lithium?
   a It is lipophilic.
   b It inhibits inositol monophosphatase in the brain.
   c It can cause alopecia.
   d The therapeutic index is low.
   e Oedema caused by lithium should not be treated with diuretics.

43 Which of the following is not a recognised side effect of the use of stimulant medication to treat ADHD?

a Hypotension

b Insomnia

c Reduction in appetite

d Development of tics

e Tachycardia

44 Which of the following is not used in the treatment of opioid dependence?

a Buprenorphine

b Lofexidine

c Methadone

d Naloxone

e Naltrexone

45 You have a patient who is about to have ECT. Which of the following medications may increase the seizure duration?

a Clozapine

b Venlafaxine

c Diazepam

d Semi-sodium valproate

e MAOIs

46 You have a patient with treatment refractory depression. Which of the following would you not consider in the first instance?

a Lithium

b High-dose venlafaxine

c Add reboxetine

d Triiodothyronine

e Tryptophan

EMIs

1 Receptors:
- a 5 HT_{1A} auto receptor
- b 5 HT_2 receptor
- c 5 HT_3 receptor
- d 5 HT transporter
- e Alpha-1 receptor
- f Alpha-2 receptor
- g GABA A receptor
- h H1 histaminergic receptor

For each pharmacological action select one receptor that is implicated in its causation.

1 Delayed therapeutic action of SSRIs

2 Nausea/vomiting due to SSRIs

3 Sedation due to tricyclic antidepressants

2 Pharmacokinetics:
- a Ionisation
- b Loading dose
- c Rate of elimination
- d Passive diffusion
- e Rate of absorption
- f Phase 1 metabolism
- g Phase 2 metabolism
- h Protein binding
- i Active transport

Which of the pharmacokinetic terms are described below?

   1 This parameter determines the duration of drug action and frequency of administration to maintain therapeutic plasma concentrations.

   2 These are conjugation reactions involving the biosynthesis of a covalent bond.

   3 This parameter depends on the rate at which the drug can pass from the gut lumen into the circulation.

3   Atypical antipsychotics:
    a Amisulpiride
    b Aripiprazole
    c Clozapine
    d Olanzapine
    e Quetiapine
    f Risperidone
    g Zotepine
    h Ziprasidone

The following is true about which atypical antipsychotic?

   1 Is available in depot formulation

   2 Has no affinity for histamine (H1) receptors

   3 Has highest affinity for $5HT_2$ receptors

   4 Requires regular blood monitoring

4   Interactions between antiepileptic drugs and other psychotropic drugs:
    a Carbamazepine
    b Phenytoin
    c Lamotrigine

d Valproate

e Gabapentin

f Vigabatrin

g Topiramate

h Ethosuximide

Which antiepileptic drug causes the following?

1 Increases level of valproate

2 Increases level of benzodiazepines

3 Level increased by lamotrigine

4 Level decreased by chronic alcohol consumption

5 Receptors:
a D3
b Alpha-2
c D1
d 5HT2
e D4
f Alpha-1
g D2
h 5HT1A
i 5HT2A

Identify the receptors involved in the therapeutic actions of the following medications:

1 Mirtazapine (2 answers)

2 Haloperidol (1 answer)

3 Clozapine (3 answers)

Answers

MCQs

1 d

(Taylor, Paton, Kerwin, pp. 120–1.)

2 c

(Taylor, Paton, Kerwin, p. 202.)

3 b

(Puri, Hall, p. 260.)

4 b

(Puri, Hall, p. 267.)

5 e

6 c

(Anderson, Reid, p. 66.)

7 e

(Puri, Hall, p. 260.)

8 b

(Anderson, Reid, p. 45.)

9 c

Amphetamine increases noradrenaline (NA) release.

10 b

11 e

(Puri, Hall, p. 266.)

12 d

(Anderson, Reid, p. 66.)

13 e

14 c

15 e

(Anderson, Reid, p. 13.)

16 a

Clozapine commonly causes constipation.

17 d

Many double-blind randomised control trials have shown fish oils are effective (Taylor, Paton, Kerwin, p. 69).

18 a

There is a randomised control trial supporting sulpiride augmentation (Taylor, Paton, Kerwin, p. 49).

19 c

(Anderson, Reid, p. 45.)

20 e

(Puri, Hall, p. 368.)

21 e

22 e

23 d

SSRIs are enzyme inhibitors of the CP450 metabolism of antipsychotics and so cause increased levels of antipsychotics.

24 c

Most psychotropic drugs are metabolised in the liver and converted from lipid-soluble to water-soluble form.

25 d

Carbamazepine and lamotrigine block sodium channels. Valproate increases the levels of GABA.

26 a

A fine tremor is a side effect of lithium, a coarse tremor occurs in toxicity (Puri, Hall, pp. 264–5).

27 e

28 a

29 d

Physical observations should be carried out frequently during the initial titration of clozapine (Taylor, Paton, Kerwin, p. 47).

30 c

Antipsychotics with a low tendency to cause weight gain include aripiprazole, haloperidol and amisulpride (Taylor, Paton, Kerwin, p. 83).

31 e

32 b

Sertraline is the drug of choice in this situation (Taylor, Paton, Kerwin, pp. 166–7).

33 d

Clozapine blood monitoring should occur weekly for 18 weeks, fortnightly for the remainder of the year and then monthly (Taylor, Paton, Kerwin, p. 65).

34 a

35 c

36 b

Phenytoin decreases clozapine levels via enzyme induction (Taylor, Paton, Kerwin, p. 48).

37 d

38 d

39 a

They are equally efficacious; the main differences are their side effects and toxicity.

40 b

41 b

Metallic taste is an acute side effect (Puri, Hall, pp. 264–5).

42 a

43 a

44 d

Naloxone is given in opioid overdose.

45 a

Clozapine is perhaps the most likely antipsychotic to increase the seizure duration (Taylor, Paton, Kerwin, p. 157).

46 c

Adding reboxetine has some evidence behind it, but is considered a second-line treatment of refractory depression (Taylor, Paton, Kerwin, pp. 150–5).

EMIs

1 1 a

   2 c

   3 h

2 1 c

   2 g

   3 e

3 1 f

   2 a

   3 f

   4 c

4 1 b

   2 d

   3 d

   4 b

5 1 b, d

   2 g

   3 c, d, e

3

Genetics

Questions

MCQs

1 Which of the following is a genetic deletion defect?
   a Rett's syndrome
   b Prader-Willi syndrome
   c Patau syndrome
   d Edward's syndrome
   e Tay-Sachs disease

2 Which of the following statements about congenital abnormalities is correct?
   a 0.5% of live newborn infants have chromosomal abnormalities.
   b The risk of an infant with Down's syndrome being born to a 20-year-old mother is 1 in 20 000.
   c 50% of foetuses have chromosomal abnormalities and the majority of these abort.
   d 1 in 400 pregnancies results in the birth of a child with a congenital abnormality.
   e 0.01% of live newborn infants have chromosomal abnormalities.

3 Which of the following is not a characteristic of fragile X syndrome?

a Macro-orchidism

b Small stature

c Prognathism

d Small low-set ears

e High-pitched perseverative speech

4 The mother of one of your patients is very concerned that her son will end up in prison like his father. Which of these statements about the genetics of antisocial behaviour is false?

a Heritability of antisocial behaviour is 40%.

b Callous-unemotional traits are highly heritable.

c Low IQ is a risk factor for offending behaviour.

d There is substantial genetic overlap between adult antisocial behaviour and alcohol and drug dependence.

e Maltreated children who have a genotype conferring high MAO-A expression are more likely to develop antisocial problems than those with low MAO-A expression.

5 Which of the following statements about alcoholism is false?

a Dopamine receptor variant DRD2 is consistently more prevalent in alcoholics than in controls.

b The concordance rate for alcoholism in male monozygotic twins is approximately 60%.

c There is a protective locus for alcoholism near the alcohol dehydrogenase gene cluster in chromosome 4.

d Linkage analysis for severe alcohol dependence has been found on chromosome 16.

e The risk of alcoholism in adopted children is more dependent on the drinking patterns of their biological parents than on those of their adoptive parents.

6 The heritability of schizophrenia is:

a 40%

b 50%

c 60%

d 70%

e 80%

7 Which of the following is false regarding microdeletions of chromosome 22q11?

   a There is an increased risk of schizophrenia.

   b It is also known as Edward's syndrome.

   c It is the second most common chromosomal abnormality.

   d It is associated with cleft lip and palate and learning disability.

   e It may include possession of the low-activity COMT Met allele.

8 In disorders with autosomal recessive transmission, which of the following is true?

   a Single heterozygotes are carriers of the abnormal trait.

   b Male offspring have a higher risk of being affected.

   c Only double heterozygotes manifest the abnormal phenotypic trait.

   d When an affected individual mates with a normal one, a quarter of the offspring will be affected.

   e When two heterozygotes mate, half the offspring will be affected.

9 In genetics, which of the following is true?

   a DNA polymerase chain reactions can amplify specific DNA fragments.

   b The lod score is not sensitive to errors in diagnosis.

   c The standard notation for gene location uses the term 'p' to indicate the long arm of the chromosome.

   d A criterion for significant genetic linkage is a lod score of less than 3.

   e Recombinant DNA is produced when plasmids are inserted into the human DNA.

10 Regarding the lod score, which option below is false?

a It is a method of assessing the likelihood of genetic linkage.

b Any multiple testing should be corrected for before interpreting the lod score.

c It is derived from the recombination fraction produced by meiosis.

d It is the common log of the odds ratio.

e Conventionally a value of -2 excludes linkage.

11 Which of the following statements about the human genome is correct?

a Mitochondrial chromosomes are identical to nuclear chromosomes.

b DNA separates its double helix in a reaction catalysed by reverse transcriptase.

c During mutation, instable complementary DNA is produced.

d In a normal human genome, about 50% of total DNA is non-coding.

e Approximately 30% to 50% of the human genome is expressed mainly in the brain.

12 Which of the following diseases and abnormal gene locations are correctly paired?

a Lesch-Nyhan syndrome: 13q 14

b Fragile X syndrome: Xp 27.3

c Huntington's disease: 3q 21.2

d Wilson's disease: 9q 12

e Friedreich's ataxia: Xq 26

13 Which of the following is true regarding twin studies?

a The concordance rate in dizygotic twins is higher than in monozygotic twins when they are born out of wedlock.

b Probandwise concordance gives lower rates than pairwise concordance.

c Taking a hospitalised sample is the best way to study twin concordance.

d The concordance rate in monozygotic twins is higher than in dizygotic twins in parental assortative mating.

e Twins have a greater risk of CNS abnormalities.

14 Which of the following does not apply to restriction fragment length polymorphisms (RFLPs)?

a They are usually bi-allelic.

b They can be produced by southern blotting.

c They allow mutations to be easily characterised.

d They are generally inherited in a simple Mendelian fashion.

e They can be used as genetic markers.

15 In disorders with autosomal dominant transmission, which of the following is incorrect?

a When one parent is homozygous, half the offspring will manifest the abnormal trait.

b When two heterozygotes mate, all the offspring will manifest the abnormal trait.

c The phenotypic trait is present in all individuals carrying the dominant allele.

d Males have a greater risk of being affected.

e When a normal individual mates with a heterozygous individual, 75% of the offspring will manifest the abnormal trait.

16 Which of the following does not apply to a gene probe?

a It can be constructed from cDNA.

b It is specifically related to the disease gene for most diseases.

c It can be constructed from mRNA.

d It has a base sequence complementary to that of a given part of a genome.

e It is a fragment of cDNA.

17 Which of the following is not a second-degree relative?

  a Grandfather

  b Aunt

  c Nephew

  d Cousin

  e Brother

18 Which of the following is not a genotype for Klinefelter syndrome?

  a XXXY

  b XXYY

  c XXX

  d XXXXY

  e XXY

19 Which of the following is an X-linked dominant disorder?

  a Rett syndrome

  b Fragile X syndrome

  c X-linked spastic paraplegia

  d Hunter syndrome

  e Cerebellar ataxia

20 Which of the following is an autosomal recessive disorder?

  a Huntington's disease

  b Acrocephalosyndactyly type I

  c Neurofibromatosis

  d Tay-Sachs disease

  e Sturge-Weber syndrome

21 Which of the following best describes the evidence regarding the role of brain-derived neurotropic factor (BDNF) in bipolar disorder?

  a There is no evidence that BDNF has a role in bipolar disorder.

b BDNF plays a role in influencing the susceptibility to bipolar disorder as a whole.

c BDNF is associated with susceptibility to the rapid cycling subset of bipolar disorder.

d BDNF is associated with susceptibility to bipolar I disorder.

e BDNF is associated with susceptibility to bipolar II disorder.

22 Which of the following statements about mitosis is incorrect?

a Telophase occurs before anaphase.

b Interphase occurs before prophase.

c Metaphase occurs after prophase.

d Metaphase occurs before anaphase.

e Prophase occurs after interphase.

23 Regarding mitochondrial mutation, which of the following is not true?

a Mitochondria are passed on from one generation to another through the cytoplasm of an egg.

b Tissues with the highest energy requirements are most affected.

c Mitochondria carry DNA molecules responsible for about 37 mitochondrial genes.

d Only females can suffer from the disorder.

e Diseases due to mitochondrial genes are passed on from the mother.

24 Regarding twin studies, which of the following is false?

a If concordance rates are high for both monozygotic and dizygotic twins, it is suggestive of a strong environmental influence.

b Concordance rate can be interpreted as an intraclass correlation.

c It is relatively easy to recruit patients.

d Bias may occur.

e Pairwise and probandwise concordance rates usually give the same results.

25 Which of the following is true regarding the familial sub-type of Alzheimer's disease?

  a The role of apoE on chromosome 19 is important.

  b Onset is usually > 60 years.

  c The presenilin-1 gene is located on chromosome 16.

  d The amyloid precursor protein gene is found on chromosome 21.

  e It has an autosomal recessive inheritance pattern.

26 Which of the following is false regarding the psychopharmacogenetics of clozapine?

  a Clozapine is primarily metabolised by CYP1A2 B.

  b Combinations of pharmacodynamic gene polymorphisms have been shown to predict response to clozapine.

  c It is unlikely to be metabolised by CYP2D6.

  d Dopamine D4 receptor polymorphisms have been shown to be strongly associated with clozapine response.

  e Response to treatment with clozapine is subject to individual variations.

27 Which of the following is seen with increasing age among genetic syndromes?

  a The behavioural phenotype is typically untreatable.

  b The skin manifestations of some conditions become more prominent.

  c The behavioural phenotype is typically static.

  d The facies of certain conditions becomes less prominent.

  e The behavioural phenotype may alter with progressive intellectual deterioration.

28 Which of the following have not been found to be associated with bipolar disorder?

  a 4p16

  b Xq24-q26

  c 21q22

d 13p12

e 16p13

29 What is the generally accepted heritability of alcoholism?

a There is little consistent evidence

b 10%

c 30%

d 50%

e 70%

30 Which of the following is false regarding the serotonin transporter-linked polymorphic region (5-HTTLPR)?

a It is an insertion/deletion polymorphism.

b It has been identified in intron 2 of the serotonin transporter gene.

c It has been associated with clinical response to SSRIs.

d It has been associated with clinical response to TCAs.

e It has been associated with response to lithium treatment.

31 Which of the following regarding recombination genetics is true?

a Lod scores are most effective for conditions with a non-Mendelian mode of inheritence.

b The value of the recombinant function varies between 0 and 1.

c Recombinant function measures the frequency of separation of alleles during meiosis.

d Linkage refers to the frequency with which two disorders are inherited concurrently.

e The closer two loci are during meiosis, the higher the chances of recombination.

32 Which of the following pathways has the greatest evidence for a genetic basis of alcoholism?

    a Serotonin

    b Dopamine

    c GABA

    d Alcohol dehydrogenase

    e Noradrenaline

33 Which of the following is a genetic disorder of carbohydrate metabolism?

    a Hartnup's disease

    b Tay-Sachs disease

    c Homocystinuria

    d Hyperlysinaemia

    e Maple syrup urine disease

34 Which of the following is a feature of *cri du chat* syndrome?

    a Deafness

    b Polydactyly

    c Gynaecomastia

    d Small hands and feet

    e Cleft lip/palate

35 Regarding Patau syndrome, which of the following is false?

    a Webbing of the neck is a feature.

    b It has an incidence of approximately one in 8000 births.

    c Polydactyly is frequent.

    d Small eyes and cataracts are features.

    e It results from trisomy 13.

36 Which of the following is not a feature of Klinefelter syndrome?

    a It is a disorder of phenotypic males.

    b Gynaecomastia.

c   Infertility is common.

d   Libido is frequently normal.

e   Congenital heart defects are common.

37   Which of the following descriptions is incorrect?

a   Transcription is a process where the gene is copied to produce an RNA molecule.

b   Epistasis is the probability that a person carrying the genotype for a dominant disease will manifest it.

c   The proteome is the complete set of proteins produced by the genome at any one time.

d   Mitosis is the process of cell division.

e   The transcriptome is the complete set of RNA transcripts produced by the genome at any one time.

38   Which of the following is not true of linkage analysis?

a   It refers to finding the rough position of disease genes relative to known genetic markers.

b   A method used is southern blotting.

c   It can only be used to study genetic disorders if the mode of inheritance is clear.

d   A method used is gene probes.

e   It can be used to study genetic disorders in families.

39   Which of these is not a difficulty with adoption studies applied to psychiatric disorders?

a   They take a long time to carry out.

b   Assortative mating may lead to a relative increase in the rate of illness in dizygotic compared to monozygotic twins.

c   The process of adoption is unlikely to be random.

d   Few cases fulfil the criteria.

e   Information about the biological father may not be available.

40 Which of the following is an autosomal recessive cause of learning disability?

a Tuberous sclerosis

b Lesch-Nyhan syndrome

c Alpert syndrome

d Galactosaemia

e Fragile X syndrome

EMIs

1 Clinical syndromes:

a Autosomal recessive inheritance

b X-linked dominant inheritance

c Trisomy 18

d Translocation between 21 and 14

e Autosomal dominant inheritance with incomplete penetrance

f Trisomy 15

g Partial deletion of the short arm of 16

h Trisomy 13

Identify a cause for the following syndromes from the list above.

1 Down's syndrome

2 Edwards' syndrome

3 Patau syndrome

2 Genetic disorders:

a Huntington gene

b Frataxin gene

c Presenelin-1

d FMRI gene

e ATP 7B gene

f Apolipoprotein E
g Hypocretin gene
h Neuregulin-1
i No gene involved

Choose a gene which is linked to the following conditions:

1 Wilson's disease

2 Early-onset Alzheimer's disease

3 Huntington's disease

4 Schizophrenia

3 Clinical features:
a A woman with a slight increase in height and a specific learning disorder
b Normal child development followed by short-lived plateau and then a rapid deterioration in motor and speech abilities
c Tall man with hypogonadism, scant facial hair and gynaecomastia
d Elfin face, peri-orbital fullness, lacy iris pattern, long philtrum and prominent lips
e An elongated face, enlarged testicles and large ears
f Transverse palmar crease, upslanting palpebral fissures and a protruding tongue
g Severe learning disability, seizures, prominent jaw and ataxic gait
h Receding jaw, wide-spaced eyes, broad nose root, occult cleft palate and external ear anomalies

Identify the clinical features from the list above which present with the following genetic abnormalities:

1 Microdeletion in chromosome 22

2 47XXY

3 Fragile X syndrome

4 Microdeletion on the long arm of chromosome 15

4 Molecular genetics:
  a A measure of how often the alleles at two loci are separated during meiotic recombination
  b Polymorphisms at restriction enzyme cleavage sites that can be used as DNA markers
  c DNA fragments are transferred from gel, where electrophoresis and DNA denaturation have taken place.
  d Crossover of genetic information between adjacent alleles
  e Cleave DNA only are locations containing specific nucleotide sequences.
  f Two genes close to each other on the same chromosome are likely to be inherited together.
  g Lengths of DNA that are constructed so that they have a nucleotide sequence complementary to that of a given part of the genome
  h A set of cloned DNA fragments representing all the genes of an organism or a given chromosome

Choose the correct description of the following techniques.

1 Gene probes

2 Southern blotting

3 Restriction fragment-length polymorphisms

Answers

MCQs

1 b

Prader-Willi is caused by a deletion of chromosome 15.

2 a

3 d

The ears are characteristically large and floppy.

4 e

It is the opposite way round. Data from the Dunedin cohort suggested that maltreated children with a genotype conferring high levels of MAO-A activity were less likely to develop antisocial problems.

5 a

6 e

Heritability is the proportion of variance attributable to genetic effects (Fear, p. 187).

7 b

It is also known as velo-cardio-facial syndrome or di George syndrome.

8 a

9 a

10 d

Lod is 'log of the odds'. It is the common log of the likelihood that the recombination fraction has a certain value.

11 e

12 b

13 e

This results from birth injuries or congenital abnormalities (Puri, Hall, p. 278).

14 c

(Puri, Hall, p. 279.)

15 b

16 b

17 e

18 c

19 a

The other options are all X-linked recessive disorders (Puri, Hall, pp. 284–5).

20 d

The other options are all autosomal dominant disorders (Puri, Hall, p. 282).

21 c

This was shown in a case-control study of over 3000 individuals from the UK. (Green K, Raybould R, Macgregor S *et al*. Genetic variation of brain-derived neurotrophic factor (BDNF) in bipolar disorder: Case-control study of over 3000 individuals from the UK. *Br J Psychiatry*. 2006; **188**: 21–5.)

22 a

Mitosis occurs via the following stages: interphase, prophase, metaphase, anaphase and telophase (Puri, Hall, p. 274).

23 d

Although mitochondrial genes are passed on from the mother, both males and females can suffer from the disorder (Leung, Passmore, p. 33).

24 e

They usually give different results (Puri, Hall, p. 278).

25 c

The presenilin-1 gene is located on chromosome 14 (Leung, Passmore, p. 39).

26 d

See Tsapakis *et al.* (Tsapakis EM, Basu A, Aitchison KJ. Clinical relevance of discoveries in psychopharmacogenetics. *Advan Psychiatr Treat.* 2004; **10**: 455–65.)

27 e

See O'Brien. (O'Brien G. Behavioural phenotypes: causes and clinical implications. *Advan Psychiatr Treat.* 2006; **12**: 338–48.)

28 d

See Craddock and Jones. (Craddock N, Jones I. Genetics of Bipolar Disorder. *J Med Genet.* 1999; **36**: 585–94.)

29 a

30 b

See Tsapakis *et al.* (Tsapakis EM, Basu A, Aitchison KJ. Clinical relevance of discoveries in psychopharmacogenetics. *Advan Psychiatr Treat.* 2004; **10**: 455–65.)

31 c

32 d

See Ball D. Genetic approaches to alcohol dependence. *Br J Psychiatry*. 2004; **185**: 449–451.

33 b

34 d

35 a

Webbing of the neck is seen in Turner's syndrome.

36 e

37 b

This is the definition of penetrance. Epistasis takes place when the action of one gene is modified by one or more others.

38 c

39 b

This is a difficulty with twin studies (Puri, Hall, p. 278).

40 d

EMIs

1 1   d

   2   c

   3   h

2 1   e

   2   c

3   a

4   h

3   1   h

2   c

3   e

4   g

4   1   g

2   c

3   b

Neurosciences

Questions

MCQs

1 Which of the following is not a limbic pathway?
   a Medial forebrain bundle
   b Dorsal longitudinal stria
   c Medial longitudinal stria
   d Stria medullaris
   e Stria terminalis

2 Which of the following is not a second messenger?
   a Cyclic AMP
   b Aspartate
   c Inositol triphosphate
   d Diacyl glycerol
   e Arachidonic acid

3 Which of the following statements about brain structures is true?

   a The striatum is made up of the caudate nucleus and the globus pallidus.

   b Basal ganglia output nuclei exert cholinergic inhibition on the thalamus.

   c The whole of the nervous system develops from the ectoderm of the embryo.

   d The pars reticulata uses dopamine as its main neurotransmitter.

   e During development, the first brain structure to myelinate is the prefrontal cortex.

4 Which of the following relationships between brain structures and functions is incorrect?

   a Amygdala: memory for emotional events

   b Limbic system activation: kindling

   c Destruction of the ventromedial hypothalamus: hyperphagia

   d Anterior hypothalamic lesion: activation of sexual activity

   e Septohippocampal system: anxiety modulation

5 In Huntington's chorea, which of the following is true?

   a The average age of onset is in the mid-twenties.

   b GAD levels are low.

   c The frontal lobes degenerate.

   d Insight is lost early.

   e The brain is of normal size.

6 Which of the following is incorrect?

a White matter changes pre-date the development of late-life depressive symptoms.

b The severity of white matter changes predicts depressive symptoms at one year.

c There is no consistent association between white matter changes and late-life depressive symptoms.

d White matter changes may be causally related to the development of late-life depressive symptoms.

e Baseline vascular burden independently predicts depression.

7 Which of the following has been suggested as a cause of Parkinsonism?

a Wilson's disease

b Mercury poisoning

c Cerebral palsy

d Lead poisoning

e Carbon monoxide poisoning

8 Which of the following is true in punch-drunk syndrome?

a The corpus callosum is perforated.

b Neuritic plaques are sometimes visible.

c Confabulation is a feature found commonly.

d Cerebral atrophy is unusual.

e The lateral ventricles are commonly enlarged.

9 Which of the following is true of cortisol levels in PTSD?

a Cortisol levels are consistently low.

b Lower cortisol levels are found in male patients compared with female patients.

c Lower cortisol levels are found in those who have suffered sexual abuse.

d Lower cortisol levels are found when measured in the morning.

e Lower cortisol levels are found in war veterans.

10 Regarding the thalamus, which is true?
    a It is part of the telencephalon.
    b The lateral geniculate nucleus receives information from the eyes.
    c The dorsomedial nucleus receives general sensation.
    d The anterior nucleus receives taste sensation.
    e It receives input from all the senses.

11 Which is the most common cerebral tumour?
    a Pituitary adenoma
    b Glioma
    c Medulloblastoma
    d Haemangioblastoma
    e Meningeal tumour

12 Which of the following neurotransmitters and peptides do not coexist?
    a Dopamine: encephalin
    b Acetylcholine: CCK (cholecystokinin)
    c Adrenaline: encephalin
    d Serotonin: TRH (thyrotrophin-releasing hormone)
    e Noradrenaline: encephalin

13 Regarding the EEG, which of the following is true?
    a Immaturity is defined as the absence of slow waves for the age.
    b Lithium can produce bursts of theta activity.
    c Electrical activity can be measured as early as 12 weeks in the human foetus.
    d Opiates produce few EEG changes when taken by addicts.
    e During aging, alpha rhythm is better preserved in men.

14 Which of the following statements regarding neuroreceptors is true?

   a 5HT3 receptors are linked to adenylate cyclase.

   b D1 receptor activation can enhance intracellular D2 receptor activity.

   c D6 receptors are predominately seen in the prefrontal cortex.

   d Stimulation of 5HT receptors increases acetylcholine release.

   e D5 receptors inhibit adenylate cyclase.

15 Which of the following is not a sign of infarction of the anterior cerebral artery?

   a Contralateral sensory loss

   b Ipsilateral Horner's syndrome

   c Clouding of consciousness

   d Ipsilateral hemiplegia

   e Aphasia

16 Which of the following inhibits the secretion of growth hormone?

   a Renal failure

   b Insomnia

   c Hepatic cirrhosis

   d Being underweight

   e Decreased fatty acids

17 Which of the following is more likely in cerebral tumours that present with psychiatric symptomatology?

   a Slow-growing tumours

   b Meningiomas

   c Infratentorial

   d Situated in the frontal lobe when associated with impairment of consciousness

   e Benign

18 Which of the following is false regarding the reticular formation?

a It is known to have connections with all of the cortex.

b It is related neurochemically to the raphe nuclei.

c It is known to cause unconsciousness during sleep.

d It is situated in the brain stem.

e It is involved in the regulation of aggression.

19 Which of the following is an example of a G-protein-coupled receptor?

a Glycine receptors

b Adrenergic receptors

c GABA type B receptors

d 5HT2 receptors

e Cholinergic receptors

20 Which of the following is true regarding thyrotropin-releasing factor (TRF)?

a It causes the release of TSH from the posterior pituitary.

b CSF levels have been found to be decreased in patients with depression.

c It causes lowering of mood when administered to normal subjects.

d Normal circadian rhythm of release is altered in depressed patients.

e When administered to depressed patients it fails to cause a normal rise in TSH levels in at least 50% of cases.

21 Which of the following is not a result of a diencephalic lesion?

a Constructional apraxia

b Akinetic mutism

c Intractable pain

d Hypersomnia

e Korsakoff's amnesia

22 Which is true regarding the neuropathology of schizophrenia?

a Gliotic reactions are often seen.

b A progressive loss of cerebral substance has been demonstrated.

c Brain weight and size are preserved.

d The hippocampus and anterior parahippocampal gyrus are particularly affected.

e The right temporal lobe is more affected than the left.

23 Regarding serotonin, which of the following is incorrect?

a L-tryptophan is a precursor.

b Storage is depleted by tetrabenazine.

c Release is dependent on sodium ions.

d Receptors of 5HT 1A subtype are located postsynaptically.

e Less than 2% of the total body serotonin is found in the central nervous system.

24 Which of the following is not a characteristic feature of punch-drunk syndrome?

a Degeneration of the substantia nigra

b Neuronal loss in the cerebral cortex and the cerebellum

c A fenestrated septum pellucidum

d Difuse cortical B-amyloid plaques

e Cortical neurofibrillary tangle formation dissimilar to Alzheimer's disease

25 Which of the following is true regarding catecholamine synthesis?

   a Dopamine is catabolised to vanillylmandelic acid.

   b Pseudocholinesterases are faster acting than true cholinesterases.

   c Tyrosine hydroxylase is involved in the biosynthesis of serotonin.

   d The conversion of noradrenaline to adrenaline involves phenylethanolamine N-methyltransferase.

   e Catechol-O-methyltransferase is not found in the liver and kidney.

26 Which of the following is a diencephalic structure?

   a Cerebellum

   b Pons

   c Pineal gland

   d Tectum

   e Medulla

27 Which of the following neurotransmitters inhibit feeding?

   a Noradrenaline

   b Serotonin

   c Galantin

   d Neuropeptide Y

   e Growth-hormone-releasing factor

28 Which of the following is true regarding cerebrospinal fluid (CSF)?

   a It passes from the fourth ventricle through the foramina of Magendie and Luschka.

   b It is formed by a passive process.

   c It is reabsorbed via an active process.

   d It is located in the subdural space.

   e Total volume is approximately 200 ml in healthy subjects.

29 Which of the following is true regarding glycine?

a It is excitatory in nature.

b It can be biosynthesized from analine.

c Receptors are blocked by strychnine.

d Release at neurones may be inhibited by tetanus toxin.

e It is found mainly in the cortex.

30 Which of the following is true regarding synaptic transmission?

a Transmission is always unidirectional in the human nervous system.

b Electrical neurotransmission is more common than chemical neurotransmission.

c Transmission occurs across a distance of approximately 25 um.

d Transmission can occur between several different areas of the surface of a neuron.

e Chemical neurotransmission is quickest.

31 Which of the following is false regarding glucocorticoids?

a They are known to be neurotoxic to the hippocampus.

b Their non-suppression by dexamethasone is a robust indicator of prognosis in depression.

c Exogenous glucocorticoids are known to cause elevation of mood.

d They directly inhibit the secretion of ACTH at the level of the hypothalamus.

e They cause psychiatric disorder in approximately 20% of patients when given in high doses.

32 Which of the following is an area of the frontal lobe?

a Supplementary motor cortex

b Primary somatosensory area

c Secondary auditory area

d Visual association area

e Wernicke's area

33 Which of the following is not part of the basal ganglia?

   a Putumen

   b Globus pallidus

   c Anterior nucleus

   d Substantia nigra

   e Red nucleus

34 Regarding the nigrostriatal pathway, which of the following is true?

   a It arises in the ventral tegmental area.

   b It may be involved in the negative symptoms of schizophrenia.

   c It passes to the neocortex, especially prefrontal areas.

   d It is concerned with sensorimotor co-coordination.

   e It passes to many components of the limbic system.

35 Which of the following is not evidence supporting the dopamine theory of schizophrenia?

   a Amphetamines increase dopamine release.

   b Disulfiram inhibits dopamine-ß-hydroxylase.

   c Monoamine reuptake inhibitors can exacerbate schizophrenia.

   d Post-mortem studies indicate increased dopamine levels in schizophrenic brains.

   e Anitpsychotics may raise HVA levels.

36 Regarding endogenous opioids, which of the following is false?

   a They are made from polypeptide precursors.

   b There are three classes of opioid receptor.

   c They are coupled to G proteins.

   d They control the release of ACTH from the anterior pituitary.

   e They have a role in addiction.

37 Which of the following is not a hormonal change found in depression?

   a Abnormal growth-hormone regulation

b Impaired osmotic regulation of vasopressin

c Blunted thyroid-stimulating hormone (TSH) response to thyrotrophin-releasing hormone (TRH) in 20–70% of patients

d Increased hypothalamic corticotrophin-releasing factor (CRF)

e Increased urinary free cortisol

38 Which of the following is secreted by the posterior pituitary?

a Oxytocin

b Growth hormone

c Prolactin

d Thyroid-stimulating hormone

e Luteinising hormone

39 Regarding cholecystokinin (CCK), which of the following is false?

a It may modulate dopaminergic-pathway activity.

b It regulates the release of bile after meals.

c It is found in high levels in the hippocampus.

d It is secreted from the hypothalamus.

e It may have a role in pain control.

40 Which of the following do not contain serotonergic nerve cells?

a The substantia nigra

b The median raphe nucleus

c The corpus callosum

d The pontomedullary region of the brain stem

e The dorsal raphe nucleus

41 Which of the following is a feature of REM sleep?

a Abolition of tendon reflexes

b Increased parasympathetic activity

c Decreased complexity of dreams

d Increased protein synthesis

e Decreased recall of dreaming

42 Which of the following statements about synaptic transmission is incorrect?

  a Amplification is an important feature of the inositol phosphate second messenger system.

  b The amount of neurotransmitter released during an action potential is related to the calcium levels at the presynaptic terminal.

  c Inhibitory postsynaptic potential results from an influx of potassium and chloride.

  d The primary structure is similar for all ion channels.

  e All postsynaptic receptors have five subunits in their general structure.

43 Which of the following areas has evidence for a role in addictive behaviours?

  a The orbitofrontal cortex

  b The hippocampus

  c The cerebellum

  d The amygdala

  e The central gyrus

44 Patients with which of the following schizophrenia symptom subgroups perform worst on mentalising tasks?

  a No disorganisation

  b Paranoid delusions

  c Auditory hallucinations

  d With disorganisation

  e In remission

45 Which of the following statements about cerebral tumours is incorrect?

  a Meningiomas grow rapidly.

  b Ependymomas spread via the cerebrospinal fluid.

  c Medulloblastomas are the most common primary tumours in childhood.

   d Acoustic neuromas affect cranial nerves V, VI, VII and VIII.

   e Adults mainly suffer from supratentorial tumours.

46 Which of the following have been associated with catatonia?
   a GABA deficiency
   b Glutamate deficiency
   c Unilateral abnormalities in metabolism in the thalamus
   d Dopamine overactivity
   e Serotonin deficiency

EMIs

1 Neuroanatomy:
   a Red nucleus
   b Mamillary bodies
   c Lentiform nucleus
   d Heschl's gyrus
   e Arcuate fasciculus
   f Olivary nucleus
   g Superior colliculus
   h Medial geniculate nucleus
   i Uncinate fasciculus

For each of the following, select the most-related neuroanatomical structure from above.

   1 Primary auditory cortex

   2 Impaired repetition of spoken word

   3 Korsakoff syndrome

2 Neurochemistry:
   a P450 enzyme inhibition
   b Effect on 5HT3 receptor
   c Effect on mesolimbic D2 receptor
   d Effect on NMDA receptor
   e P450 enzyme induction
   f Effect on 5HT2 receptor
   g Effect on D2 tuberoinfundibular receptor
   h Effect on nigrostriatal D2 receptor
   i Effect on alpha 1-adrenoreceptor

Select one of the above that is the mechanism by which each of these scenarios occur.

   1 A woman taking sertraline is commenced on amitriptyline. She becomes confused and agitated and exhibits myoclonus.

   2 A woman taking St John's wort becomes pregnant despite taking the oral contraceptive pill.

   3 A patient taking antipsychotics develops EPSE.

3 Neuropathology:
   a Status spongiosus
   b Lewy bodies
   c Copper deposits in the basal ganglia
   d Hirano bodies
   e Zebra cells
   f Reduced hippocampal volume
   g Cellular degeneration of the substantia nigra
   h Reduced cerebral aluminium levels
   i B-cells in the mamillary bodies
   j Neurofibrillary tangles
   k Circumscribed frontal atrophy

l Medial temporal structures sparing

m Generalised cortical atrophy

Identify the most relevant associated neuropathological changes for the following disorders.

1 Parkinson's disease (2 answers)

2 Creutzfeldt-Jakob disease

3 Alzheimer's disease (3 answers)

4 Pick's disease

5 Lewy body dementia (2 answers)

4 Functions of neurons:
   a Microglia
   b Schwann cells
   c Oligodendrocytes
   d Astrocytes
   e Purkinje cells
   f Chandelier cells
   g Pyramidal neuron
   h Martinotti cells
   i Double bouquet cells

Choose from the list above functions that:

1 Are involved in removing dead tissue from the nervous system (2 answers)

2 Mainly use glutamate as their neurotransmitter

3 Are involved in repair of the myelin sheath of axons (2 answers)

Answers

MCQs

1 b

The dorsal longitudinal fasicularis is a limbic pathway (Puri, Hall, p. 179).

2 b

Aspartate is an excitory amino acid (Leung, Passmore, p. 120).

3 d

4 d

Anterior hypothalamic lesions are associated with inhibition of sexual activity.

5 c

(Puri, Hall, p. 553.)

6 c

See the longitudinal study by Tedorczuk *et al.* (Teodorczuk A, O'Brien JT, Firbank MJ *et al.* White matter changes and late-life depressive symptoms: longitudinal study. *Br J Psychiatry.* 2007; **191**: 212–7.)

7 e

Carbon monoxide poisoning has been suggested in causing Parkinsonism.

8 d

Cerebral atrophy is common.

9 c

See Meewisse *et al.* for a systematic review and meta-analysis. (Meewisse M-L, Reitsma JB, De Vries G-J *et al.* Cortisol and post-traumatic stress disorder in adults: systematic review and meta-analysis. *Br J Pychiatry.* 2007; **191**: 387–92.)

10 c

(Fear, p. 122.)

11 b

(Puri, Hall, pp. 196–7.)

12 b

Acetylcholine and VIP (vasoactive intestinal polypeptide) coexist.

13 d

(Puri, Hall, pp. 222–3.)

14 b

15 d

Contralateral hemiplegia is a sign.

16 b

17 d

18 e

19 a

20 d

21 a

This is usually a result of a parietal lobe lesion.

22 d

Reduced cell number and abnormal cellular arrangement are evident in the hippocampus and entorhinal cortex.

23 c

Release is dependent on calcium ions.

24 e

The cortical neurofibrillary tangle formation is similar to that of Alzheimer's disease.

25 d

26 c

(Fear, p. 122.)

27 b

This is a common side effect of SSRIs, and fluoxetine is licenced for the treatment of bulimia nervosa. All the other options stimulate feeding.

28 a

29 c

30 d

31 d

ACTH is secreted by the pituitary and so reduction of ACTH secretion by the hypothalamus is indirect.

32 a

(Leung, Passmore, pp. 95–7.)

33 c

The anterior nucleus is part of the thalamus.

34 d

(Leung, Passmore, p. 111.)

35 e

(Puri, Hall, p. 376.)

36 d

This is a role of cortictrophin-releasing hormone (CRH) (Leung, Passmore, p. 128).

37 b

This is found in anorexia nervosa (Leung, Passmore, p. 160).

38 a

All the other options are secreted by the anterior pituitary (Leung, Passmore, p. 158).

39 d

CRH is secreted from the hypothalamus.

40 c

41 d

(Puri, Hall, p. 221.)

42 a

Amplification is an important feature of the adenate cyclase system.

43 a

See the systematic review by Dom *et al.* (Dom G, Sabbe B, Hulstijn W *et al.* Substance use disorders and the orbitofrontal cortex: systematic review of behavioural decision-making and neuroimaging studies. *Br J Psychiatry*. 2005; **187**: 209–20.)

44 d

See meta-analysis by Sprong *et al.* (Sprong M, Schothorst P, Vos E *et al.* Theory of mind in schizophrenia: meta-analysis. *Br J Psychiatry*. 2007; **191**: 5–13.)

45 a

Meningiomas are usually slow growing.

46 a

See Rajagopal. (Rajagopal S. Catatonia. *Advan Psychiatr Treat.* 2007; **13**: 51–9.)

EMIs

1 1 d

   2 e

   3 b

2 1 f

   2 e

   3 h

3 1 b, g

   2 a

   3 d, j, m

   4 k

   5 b, l

4 1 a, d

   2 g

   3 b, c

Advanced psychological processes and treatments

Questions

MCQs

1 Which of the following is not one of Beck's cognitive distortions?
   a Selective abstraction
   b Dichotomous thinking
   c Overgeneralisation
   d Arbitrary inference
   e Worthlessness

2 Which of the following is a technique using the principles of classical conditioning?
   a Functional analysis
   b Systematic desensitisation
   c Modelling
   d Biofeedback
   e Chaining

3 Which of the following is not a function of the prefrontal cortex?

   a Problem solving

   b Verbal regulation

   c Tertiary level of motor control

   d Expressive speech

   e Programming and planning of sequences of behaviour

4 Which of the following is not a core skill in dialectical behavioural therapy?

   a Therapeutic alliance

   b Mindfulness

   c Stress tolerance

   d Interpersonal effectiveness

   e Emotional regulation

5 What was the main finding of the Adolescent Depression Antidepressant and Psychotherapy Trial (ADAPT)?

   a Family therapy is effective in treating depression in adolescents.

   b Cognitive-behavioural therapy and an SSRI are no better than an SSRI alone.

   c Cognitive-behavioural therapy is better than routine care.

   d Cognitive-behavioural therapy and an SSRI are better than an SSRI alone.

   e Family therapy is better than routine care.

6 Which of the following is not a recommended initial treatment for mild depression in primary care?

   a Watchful waiting

   b Computerised CBT

   c Exercise

   d SSRIs

   e Guided self-help

7 Regarding the 'sick role' as described by Parsons, which of the following is false?

a The individual sufferer may be expected not to complete normal activities and responsibilities.

b The individual is regarded as being in need of care and unable to get better by his or her decision and will.

c The individual may adopt the role as a permanent state if he or she has a chronic illness.

d The individual must want to get well as soon as possible.

e The individual should seek professional advice and cooperate with the doctor.

8 Which of the following is true regarding cognitive behavioural therapy with older adults?

a It does not make reference to the patient's early life experiences.

b It may involve other family members.

c It is known to be equally effective with different subtypes of depression.

d It is not a suitable treatment when depression arises from actual life problems.

e It is less effective in the treatment of depressive illness than it is with younger adults.

9 Which of the following is an application of classical conditioning?

a Token economy

b Biofeedback

c Punishment techniques

d Star charts

e Systemic desensitisation

10 Which of these statements about the treatment of alcoholism is incorrect?

a Motivational enhancement therapy involves the patient developing the solution for his or her alcohol problems through his or her own resources.

b CBT involves developing strategies to deal with high risk situations when the patient may want to drink.

c There is no evidence for the effectiveness of Alcoholics Anonymous and related 12-step programmes.

d The major determinant of abstinence after 1 year is the initial treatment, with inpatient detoxification being superior to outpatient detoxification.

e Brief interventions by primary healthcare providers have been shown to reduce drinking levels.

11 A 67-year-old man presents with gradual memory loss. What test could you perform to obtain an estimate of his pre-morbid IQ?

a Stroop test

b National Adult Reading Test

c Weschler Memory Scale

d Mini Mental State Examination

e Wisconsin Card Sorting Test

12 Which of the following is not an experiential-expressive therapy?

a Dialectical behavioural therapy

b Client-centred therapy

c Gestalt therapy

d Counselling

e Supportive psychotherapy

13 Which of the following personality disorders is incorrectly paired with the DSM-IV cluster?

a Paranoid: cluster A

b Dependent: cluster C

c Histrionic: cluster B

d Schizoid: cluster C

e Borderline: cluster B

14 Which of the following is incorrect regarding cognitive behavioural techniques?

a They cannot be applied with patients suffering from dementia.

b They are primarily aimed at enabling depressed or anxious patients to think more positively.

c They need to be modified for use with older patients.

d They can be employed by therapists without full CBT training.

e They include the 'three column technique'.

15 Which of the following psychological interventions is recommended in schizophrenia?

a Psychodynamic psychotherapy

b Counselling

c Behavioural family therapy

d Supportive psychotherapy

e Interpersonal therapy

16 Which of the following did the SoCRATES study not show?

a All groups had a significant improvement on the PANSS at 18 months.

b There were no significant overall differences in the outcomes of patients between CBT and supportive counselling.

c Hallucinations improved more with CBT than with supportive counselling.

d Those receiving a psychological therapy improved quicker than those receiving treatment as usual.

e Social functioning improved more with supportive counselling compared with CBT.

17 Which of the following is false in relation to attitude change?

a Low self-esteem and intelligence of the recipient increases the likelihood that complex communications will be persuasive.

b Message repetition can be a persuasive influence.

c Interactive personal discussions are more persuasive than mass-media communication.

d Implicit messages are more persuasive for the more intelligent recipient.

e Attractive people are more persuasive communicators.

18 Which of the following is a term to describe being unable to recognise familiar faces?

a Prosopagnosia

b Agraphaesthesia

c Astereognosia

d Autotopagnosia

e Hemisomatognosis

19 Which of the following is not a test of memory?

a Rey-Osterrieth Test

b Boston Naming Test

c WMS-R

d Benton Visual Retention Test

e Paired associate learning test

20 NICE have reviewed computerised CBT packages. Which of the following statements is correct?

a They have recommended a package for patients with OCD.

b All packages were found to be effective in the treatment of depression.

c A package was recommended for the treatment of panic and phobia.

d Cost-effectiveness was not considered.

e It was recommended that those currently using packages for OCD should stop.

21 Regarding compulsions in OCD, which of the following is true?

   a They can be resisted by focusing attention inwards on subjective feelings.

   b They are entirely voluntary.

   c They cannot be mental acts.

   d They can lead to psychosis if left untreated.

   e They may initially function as a means of avoiding anxiety.

22 A 58-year-old man presents with a year-long history of progressive personality change. An MRI scan shows a large meningioma compressing the prefrontal cortex on the left. Which test result is most likely to be impaired?

   a Stroop test

   b National Adult Reading Test

   c Weschler Memory Scale

   d Mini Mental State Examination

   e Wisconsin Card Sorting Test

23 Which of the following is an application of operant conditioning?

   a Systemic desensitisation

   b Flooding

   c Star charts

   d Aversion therapy

   e Use of enuresis alarm

24 Which of the following is a cognitive process in OCD?

   a Finishing a washing ritual when hands are clean

   b Underestimation of the likelihood of harm

   c Tolerance of uncertainty

   d Overinflated sense of responsibility for harm

   e Thought-action dissociation

25 Which of the following statements about the evidence for dialectical
    behavioural therapy in patients with borderline personality disorder
    and self-harm is correct?

    a It is superior to CBT and treatment as usual at one-year
       follow-up.

    b It has no effect on incidence of self-harm.

    c It is of comparable efficacy to CBT.

    d There is no benefit compared to treatment as usual.

    e It has no effect on the number of inpatient admissions.

26 Which of the following is not one of the primary mental abilities
    as described by Thurstone (1938)?

    a Verbal relations

    b Perpetual speed

    c Broad auditory perception

    d Memory

    e Word fluency

27 Which of the following is a performance subtest of the Wechsler
    Adult Intelligence Scale (WAIS-III)?

    a Block design

    b Vocabulary

    c Arithmetic

    d Digit span

    e Information

28 Which of the following fears has the highest prevalence in the nor-
    mal population?

    a Water

    b Public transport

    c Closed spaces

    d Heights

    e Storms

29 Which of the following is a humanistic theory of motivation?

a Homeostatic drive theory (Cannon, 1929)

b Needs theory (McClelland, 1985)

c Hierarchy of needs (Maslow, 1943)

d Drive reduction theory (Hull, 1943)

e Arousal reduction theory (Hebb, 1949)

30 The Tower of London test (Shallice, 1982) assesses the ability of which executive function?

a Set shifting

b Planning

c Inhibition

d Working memory

e Fluency

31 Which of the following is a feature of long-term memory?

a Mainly echoic or visual modality

b Prefrontal brain structures are involved

c Retention of information is by maintenance rehearsal

d Limbic structures are involved

e Tested by digit span

32 Which of the following is not a type of social power as described by Collins and Raven (1969)?

a Reward power

b Coercive power

c Position power

d Informational power

e Expert power

33 Which of the following is not true of the Minnesota Multiphasic Personality Inventory (MMPI)?

a It is a 566-item true/false test.

b It has 10 clinical scales.

c It can be used to measure psychopathy.

d It contains four validity scales.

e It can be used to produce a DSM-IV diagnosis.

34 Which of the following is not a primary emotion as described by Plutchik?

a Disgust

b Elation

c Acceptance

d Anticipation

e Anger

35 Which of the following is not associated with Type A personality?

a Increased systolic blood pressure

b Increased plasma cortisol

c Increased occipital alpha activity on EEG

d Increased heart rate

e Increased plasma adrenaline

36 Which of the following is not a feature of cognitive analytic therapy (CAT)?

a It was developed by Anthony Ryle in 1990.

b The procedural sequence model is a key concept.

c Sessions are usually for 6–12 months.

d A goodbye letter is usually written.

e *Dilemmas*, *snags* and *traps* are the three essential patterns of neurotic repetitions.

37 Which of the following is not a cognitive distortion as recognised in CBT?

 a Arbitrary inference

 b Magnification/minimisation

 c Selective abstraction

 d Overgeneralisation

 e Striving for superiority

38 Regarding the personal construct theory, which of the following is false?

 a It led to the development of the repertory grid.

 b It suggests that personality is the sum of a cluster of neurotic complexes.

 c It emphasises man as a scientist.

 d It suggests that people may sacrifice themselves to preserve core constructs.

 e It incorporates theories on creativity.

39 Which of the following is true when judgements about visual measurements are expressed?

 a A unanimous group of 20 is much more likely than a unanimous group of three to persuade an individual to change his or her decision.

 b The majority of individuals will stick to their own opinion in the face of group opposition.

 c An individual will usually stick with his or her original decision if the group he or she is in express a contrary opinion.

 d An individual is far less likely to yield to a group decision if just one other individual agrees with him or her.

 e An individual can easily persuade a group to change their group decision.

40 Which of the following is not a behavioural therapy technique?

   a Aversive conditioning

   b Modelling

   c Positive reappraisal

   d Contingency management

   e Flooding

41 Which of the following psychoanalysts is correctly paired with their area of psychotherapy?

   a Bion: group psychotherapy

   b Moreno: psychodrama

   c Janov: primal therapy

   d Winnicott: child analysis

   e Perls: couple therapy

42 Which psychoanalyst argued that libido was not just a sexual instinct but a more general life force that includes an innate drive for creativity?

   a Carl Jung

   b Sigmond Freud

   c Melanie Klein

   d Alfred Adler

   e Karen Horney

43 Which of the following is true of the Bedford method of assessing life events?

   a It rates life events on a severity scale of 1–100.

   b It takes into account how the individual felt about the event.

   c It is a self-rating questionnaire.

   d It allows both idiographic and nomothetic information to be combined.

   e It rates events independently of their context.

44 Which of the following is true regarding the Parental Bonding Instrument?

  a It measures dependency.

  b It yields abnormal care scores from neurotic depressives.

  c It is based on a two-hour interview.

  d It measures bonding from the parents' viewpoint.

  e It yields normal control scores from neurotic depressives.

45 Which of the following is not true when testing disturbances of information processing?

  a Short-term recall memory deficits occur in schizophrenia.

  b The Continuous Performance Test (CPT) involves the presentation of target stimuli amongst random stimuli on a computer screen.

  c Smooth pursuit eye movement is abnormal in 80% of first-degree relatives with schizophrenia.

  d A pendulum can be used to test smooth pursuit eye movement.

  e There are deficits in conceptual shifts in chronic schizophrenia.

EMIs

1 Defence mechanisms:

a Splitting

b Projective identification

c Denial

d Sublimation

e Repression

f Reaction formation

g Displacement

h Regression

i Introjection

j Intellectualisation

k Suppression

l Altruism

Which defence mechanisms are described in the following scenarios?

1 An 11-year-old boy, whose mother recently died in a car accident, has been bed-wetting and has started sucking his thumb.

2 A woman whose husband has been diagnosed with motor neurone disease addresses a support group and says she paints in order to help her deal with her stress.

3 A young female inpatient makes a complaint about the nursing staff to her doctor, who she feels can help her because he is the best doctor she has ever had.

4 A patient is very agitated and is insisting on being discharged. The doctor assessing her is left feeling extremely anxious about discharging her, and the patient now seems very calm.

5 A patient tells of how happy her childhood was and how her mother was wonderful until she had to give her up for financial

reasons. From the notes it is clear that she was taken into care because of severe neglect by her mother.

2 Psychotherapy techniques:
   a Supportive psychotherapy
   b Dialectical behaviour therapy
   c Flooding
   d Exposure and response prevention
   e Jacobson's progressive muscular relaxation
   f Thought stopping
   g Systemic therapy
   h Cognitive analytical therapy
   i Psychodynamic psychotherapy

Which techniques would be most appropriate in the following situations?

   1 A 25-year-old woman, having recently split up from her boyfriend, presents to A & E with several cuts on her wrists, complaining of feeling empty inside. She has a past history of unstable relationships and self-harm.

   2 A 32-year-old woman who feels anxious all the time

   3 A 21-year-old man who has obsessive compulsive disorder (2 answers)

3 Therapists:
   a Freud
   b Klein
   c Adler
   d Winnicott
   e Beck
   f Jung
   g Ellis
   h Rogers

Which therapist is associated with the following techniques?

1 Interpretation of the transference

2 Play therapy

3 Unconditional positive regard for the patient

4 Elicitation of underlying dysfunctional assumptions

4 Psychological treatment:
  a Diary keeping
  b Goodbye letter
  c Role transitions
  d Free association
  e Parapraxis
  f Homework
  g Lying on a couch
  h Time limited
  i Procedural sequence model

For each of the following therapies choose the most appropriate features:

1 Cognitive analytic therapy (3 answers)

2 Psychodynamic psychotherapy (3 answers)

3 Interpersonal therapy (2 answers)

Answers

MCQs

1 e

2 b

Functional analysis and chaining use the principles of operant conditioning (Puri, Hall, p. 7).

3 d

Expressive speech is a function of Broca's area, which is not in the prefrontal cortex (Puri, Hall, p. 60).

4 a

The therapeutic alliance is not one of the core skills that are central to the process of dialectical behavioural therapy.

5 b

The ADAPT study was a randomised control trial considering the use of SSRIs with or without CBT in adolescents with depression. It showed no additional benefit to adding CBT to SSRIs. (Goodyer I, Dubicka B, Wilkinson P *et al*. Selective serotonin reuptake inhibitors (SSRIs) and routine specialist care with and without cognitive behaviour therapy in adolescents with major depression: randomised controlled trial. *BMJ*. 2007; **335**: 142–50.)

6 d

National Institute for Health and Clinical Excellence. *Depression: NICE guideline 23*. London: NIHCE; 2004.

7 c

Parsons viewed the sick role as temporary. Those with chronic illness are not expected to occupy the sick role permanently, but at time of exacerbations of illness.

8 b

Patients often wish to tackle relationship problems with other family members. Family members can help as co-therapists.

9 e

All the other options are applications of operant conditioning.

10 c

Project MATCH was a large multi-centre trial that found some advantages to the 12-step programme compared with CBT and motivational interviewing.

11 b

12 a

(Johnstone, Cunningham-Owens, Lawrie *et al.*, p. 311.)

13 d

Schizoid personality disorder is in cluster A of DSM-IV.

14 b

The primary aim of CBT in depression is to facilitate identification of negative thinking so that logical errors and bias can be reduced.

15 c

Family interventions in schizophrenia are recommended by NICE (National Institute for Clinical Excellence. Schizophrenia: NICE guideline 1. London: NICE; 2002).

16 e

SoCRATES study. (Lewis S, Tarrier N, Haddock G *et al.* Randomised controlled trial of cognitive-behavioural therapy in early schizophrenia: acute-phase outcomes. *Br J Psychiatry.* 2002; **181**: s91–7.)

17 a

It is the opposite (Puri, Hall, p. 50).

18 a

19 b

The Boston Naming Test is a language test (Puri, Hall, pp. 93–6).

20 c

National Institute for Health and Clinical Excellence. *Depression and Anxiety – Computerised Cognitive Behavioural Therapy (CCBT): NICE technology appraisal 97.* London: NIHCE; 2006.

21 e

Veale D. Cognitive-behavioural therapy for obsessive-compulsive disorder. *Advan Psychiatr Treat.* 2007; **13**: 438–46.

22 e

23 c

The other options are all applications of classical conditioning.

24 d

Veale D. Cognitive–behavioural therapy for obsessive–compulsive disorder. *Advan Psychiatr Treat.* 2007; **13**: 438–46.

25 a

Linehan demonstrated in a randomised control trial that for patients with borderline personality disorder and self-harm DBT was superior at 1-year follow-up compared to CBT or treatment as usual. (Linehan M, Heard HL, Armstrong HE. Naturalistic follow-up of a behavioral treatment for chronically parasuicidal borderline patients. *Arch Gen Psychiatry.* 1993; **50**: 971–4.)

26 c

Thurstone described 7 primary mental abilities. Broad auditory perception is part of the *three-stratum model* of intelligence as described by Carroll.

27 a

The other options are all verbal subtests.

28 d

18.4% of the normal population have a fear of heights (Eaton WW, Kessler LG. *Epidemiologic field methods in psychiatry: the NIMH Epidemiologic Catchment Area Program.* Orlando, Fla.: Academic Press; 1985.).

29 c

The remaining are either biopsychological or sociopsychological approaches.

30 b

The Tower of Hanoi test can also be used.

31 d

The other options are all features of short-term (working) memory.

32 c

33 e

34 b

35 c

Type A personality is associated with reduced occipital alpha activity on EEG.

36 c

CAT usually takes 10 to 12 sessions.

37 e

Striving for superiority was described by Alfred Adler and refers to personality development.

38 b

As reported by Asch in 1955.

39 d

40 c

Positive reappraisal is an emotion-focused coping method.

41 e

Perls is associated with Gestalt therapy.

42 a

Jung also suggested that people develop, over time, differing degrees of introversion or extraversion.

43 d

Unlike many life-event scales and schedules, the Bedford College method takes into account the social context of that event in measuring the impact on the individual.

44 e

The Parental Bonding Instrument is a 25-item questionnaire given to patients who rate statements about their mother or father. Neurotic depressives give lower care scores and higher control scores to their parents.

45 c

Smooth pursuit eye movement is abnormal in approximately 50% of first-degree relatives with schizophrenia.

EMIs

1 1 h

2 d

3 a

4 b

5 f

2 1 b

2 e

3 d, f

3 1 a

2 b

3 h

4 e

4 1 b, h, i

2 d, e, g

3 c, h

6

Epidemiology

Questions

MCQs

1 Regarding the epidemiology of sexual disorders, which of the following is false?

 a Sexual problems at the start of a marriage are associated with a high rate of divorce.

 b Impotence occurs in 10% of 40-year-olds.

 c Sexual problems in men are mainly due to erectile dysfunction.

 d Sexual problems and marital difficulties occur in approximately 5% of psychiatric clinic attendees.

 e Sexual problems are reported more often by men than by women.

2 You are advising one of your patients about the association between cannabis and schizophrenia. Which of the following statements best reflects the evidence?

 a There is no association between cannabis and schizophrenia.

 b Cannabis reduces the risk of developing schizophrenia.

 c Cannabis leads to a twofold increased risk of developing schizophrenia.

 d Cannabis leads to a threefold increased risk of developing schizophrenia.

 e Cannabis leads to a fourfold increased risk of developing schizophrenia.

3 Which of the following is true of semi-structured interviews?

a The questions are prescriptive and uniform.

b Responses may be restricted to several categories.

c Relatively little training is needed for interviewers.

d They usually result in qualitative analysis.

e They allow easy data analysis.

4 Which of the following is false regarding the epidemiology of mood disorders?

a There is a raised incidence in those who are not married.

b The point prevalence of depressive symptoms is over 30%.

c The average age of onset of depressive episodes is in the late thirties.

d The lifetime risk of developing bipolar disorder is 0.6–1.1%.

e There are problems in comparing epidemiological studies because of the use of differing diagnostic criteria.

5 Which of the following tests is self-rated?

a Present State Examination (PSE)

b Structured Clinical Interview for DSM-IV (SCID)

c General Health Questionnaire (GHQ)

d Halstead Reitan Battery

e Composite International Diagnostic Interview (CIDI)

6 Which of the following is the most important confounding factor in calculating morbidity and mortality rates in epidemiological studies?

a Gender

b Age

c Social class

d Ethnicity

e Population size

7 Every week in the UK how many of the 16–65-year-old population have suicidal ideation?

a 0.01%

b 0.1%

c 1%

d 5%

e 10%

8 Which of the following statements about incidence and prevalence is true?

a The incidence of a disease is related to its duration.

b Cross-sectional studies measure incidence.

c Catch-recatch methods are used to assess incidence.

d Case-control studies provide information about incidence of a disorder.

e A chronic condition will have a low prevalence and a high incidence.

9 What does the evidence suggest about the variation in incidence of psychoses in the UK in terms of ethnicity?

a There is no variation in terms of ethnicity.

b The incidence is higher in the host population.

c Psychoses are twice as common in the black and ethnic minority groups.

d The incidence is lower in migrants.

e Psychoses are three times as common in the black and ethnic minority groups.

10 Regarding the epidemiology of sleep disorders, which of the following is false?

a The estimated prevalence of insomnia in adults ranges from 15% to over 40%.

b Somnambulism occurs at least once in 15% of children aged 5–12 years.

c Insomnia is less prevalent in the elderly.

d Night terrors occur on a frequent basis in 1–4% of children.

e Daytime drowsiness occurs in 0.35–4% of the population.

11 The mother of one of your patients with schizophrenia is concerned about the stories she has read in the newspapers about schizophrenics killing people. How many perpetrators of homicide have schizophrenia?

a 0.1%

b 0.5%

c 1%

d 5%

e 10%

12 Which of the following is not an index of alcohol consumption?

a Liver cirrhosis mortality

b Arrests for drink-driving

c Arrests for rape

d Cases of assault and battery

e Deaths from alcohol poisoning

13 Regarding the epidemiology of delusional disorders, which of the following is false?

a Males have a higher risk than females.

b Sufferers are often unmarried.

c There is a point prevalence of 0.03%.

d There is often a history of long-standing personality disorders.

e The mean age of onset for males is 35.

14 Regarding the sex difference in schizophrenia, which of the following is false?

a Males have an earlier age of onset.

b Males are more likely to express negative symptoms.

c Males have a higher rate of structural brain abnormalities.

d Males are more likely to have had abnormal premorbid intellectual and social functioning.

e Males have fewer relapses.

15 Regarding the epidemiology of eating disorders, which of the following is false?

a The EAT questionnaire has been shown to have good validity in the clinical setting.

b Patients with anorexia nervosa tend to avoid participating in surveys.

c Different countries have similar prevalence rates.

d A point prevalence of 4–5% exists for young British women.

e Anorexia nervosa has increased in recent decades.

16 Regarding the epidemiology of personality disorders, which of the following is true?

a The community prevalence of paranoid personality disorder is 5%.

b The male to female sex ratio of antisocial personality disorder is 7:1.

c The outpatient prevalence of borderline personality disorder is 20%.

d Obsessive-compulsive personality disorder is the most frequently reported.

e The ECQ study found a prevalence of personality disorder in the community of 12%.

17 Which of the following has been found in epidemiological studies?

   a Heavy alcohol consumption is consistently associated with later dementia.

   b Men with schizophrenia tend to have more affective symptoms than women do.

   c Prevalence rates for schizophrenia are stable across temporal and geographical boundaries.

   d Head injury is associated with later dementia.

   e The association between depression and family history of depression increases with age.

18 Which of the following is true when measuring morbidity?

   a The average duration of sickness is the incidence rate divided by the point prevalence.

   b Incidence is best studied using a longitudinal survey.

   c The incidence rate is the number of completed episodes of illness in a year.

   d A crude rate relates to particular sections of the population.

   e The point prevalence rate is the number of illnesses at any time over the number of people exposed to risk in a period.

19 Which of the following is false regarding the epidemiology of child and adolescent disorders?

   a The point prevalence of conduct disorder amongst 10- and 11-year-olds is approximately 4%.

   b The incidence of ADHD decreases with increasing age.

   c There is an equal sex ratio for elective mutism.

   d The prevalence of non-organic enuresis in 7-year-old boys is approximately 7%.

   e There is an equal sex ratio for Tourette's syndrome.

20 Regarding the epidemiology of premenstrual syndrome, which of the following is not true?

   a 40% of women experience some cyclical premenstrual symptoms.

   b Prevalence decreases with increasing parity.

   c There is a higher prevalence in those around 30 years of age.

   d Women using oral contraceptives have reduced rates of premenstrual symptoms.

   e 2–10% of women report severe premenstrual symptoms.

21 The definition of period prevalence is:

   a The rate of occurrence of new cases of a disease in a defined population over a given period of time

   b The proportion of a defined population that has a given disease at a given point in time

   c The proportion of a defined population that has or has had a disease at a given point in time

   d The proportion of live births that has a given disease

   e The proportion of a defined population that has a given disease during a given interval of time

22 Which of the following is a semi-structured interview?

   a General Health Questionnaire (GHQ)

   b Edinburgh Postnatal Depression Scale

   c Halstead Reitan Battery

   d Beck's Depression Inventory (BDI)

   e Schedule for Clinical Assessment in Neuropsychiatry (SCAN)

23 Schizophrenic births in the winter/spring account for what percentage excess?

   a 1–3%

   b 2–5%

   c 5–8%

   d 9–12%

   e 13–16%

24 Which of the following is not associated with the development of depression in adults?

a Loneliness

b Male gender

c Loss of mother in early life

d Bereavement

e Smoking

25 Regarding immigrants, which of the following is not true?

a Immigrants from the West Indies have been found to have a higher prevalence of schizophrenia compared to the British-born black population.

b Immigrants who are refugees have a lower psychiatric morbidity because they have a positive view of their new surroundings.

c Immigrants face a cultural shock, as defined by Toffler (1970).

d Immigrants undergo a process of acculturation.

e Immigrants who are settlers tend to take a positive view of their new surroundings.

26 People in which occupation have the highest rate of alcohol dependency?

a Bus drivers

b Receptionists

c Clergymen

d Dentists

e Teachers

27 Which of the following is associated with school refusal?

a It is more common in males.

b The most common age is approximately 11 years.

c Younger children have a better prognosis.

d It is associated with the lower social classes.

e In younger children the most common cause is depression.

28 Which of the following is false?

   a Case series can provide useful information on rare diseases.

   b Studies of disease frequency require a control group.

   c Qualitative studies do not require a control group.

   d Correlational studies are prone to the ecological fallacy.

   e Case report findings can always be attributable to chance.

29 Regarding the epidemiology of heroin misuse, which of the following is not true?

   a The number of addicts notified to the Home Office has increased dramatically over the last 30 years.

   b Polydrug use has increased significantly.

   c Most heroin users are aged between 20 and 30 years.

   d The male to female ratio is 2:1.

   e Youth culture has become more rejecting of heroin use in recent years.

30 Which of the following was found in the Epidemiological Catchment Area study?

   a A 6-month prevalence for agoraphobia of 6–8%

   b A 6-month prevalence for simple phobia of 12–16%

   c A 6-month prevalence for social phobia of 0.5–1%

   d A 6-month prevalence for experiencing a panic attack of 3%

   e A 6-month prevalence for generalised anxiety disorder of 7–10%

31 What is the prevalence of neurotic disorders among adults in the UK?

   a 1 in 20

   b 1 in 15

   c 1 in 10

   d 1 in 6

   e 1 in 4

32 For which of the following months of birth is there evidence that there is an increased risk of suicide?

a May

b January

c September

d December

e August

33 Regarding the epidemiology of OCD, which of the following is true?

a Females have a higher incidence than males.

b There is a peak age of onset of 30 years.

c The lifetime prevalence rate is approximately 5%.

d Rutter found no cases among 2000 10- and 11-year-olds on the Isle of Wight.

e The six-month prevalence is less than 1%.

34 Which of the following data is not required to calculate disability-adjusted life years (DALYs) for a disease?

a Standardised mortality ratio

b Incidence

c Impact on health

d Prevalence

e Impact on life expectancy

35 When female alcoholics are compared to male alcoholics, which of the following is false?

a Females commit fewer antisocial acts when intoxicated.

b Females are more susceptible to liver cirrhosis.

c Females more often drink alone.

d Females make more suicide attempts.

e Females have a family history of alcoholism less often.

36 Regarding exhibitionism, which of the following is true?

   a Greater than 15% of offenders have a learning disability.

   b Cyproterone acetate is the treatment of choice for the recidivist offender.

   c It is the most frequent parasexual activity subject to prosecution.

   d Exposure is usually a prelude to rape.

   e The offenders are characteristically aged more than 50 years.

EMIs

1 Screening:

   a Post-test odds

   b Positive predictive value

   c Negative likelihood ratio

   d Specificity

   e Negative predictive value

   f Positive likelihood ratio

   g Pre-test odds

   h Sensitivity

Match the following definitions with the terms above.

   1 The proportion of people with the disease who will test positive with the screening test

   2 The proportion of those scoring negative on the test who will not actually have the disease

   3 The proportion of people without the disease who will test negative with the screening test

   4 The decrease in the odds of having a disease when the test result is negative

2   Measuring psychiatric disorder:
   a Hamilton Rating Scale for Depression (HDRS)
   b Present State Examination (PSE)
   c Structured Clinical Interview for DSM-IV (SCID)
   d General Health Questionnaire (GHQ)
   e Edinburgh Postnatal Depression Scale
   f Halstead Reitan Battery
   g Montgomery-Ashberg Depression Rating Scale (MADRS)
   h Composite International Diagnostic Interview (CIDI)
   i Beck's Depression Inventory (BDI)
   j Schedule for Clinical Assessment in Neuropsychiatry (SCAN)

Which of the measures above are:

   1 Self-rated (3 answers)

   2 Semi-structured interviews (3 answers)

Answers

MCQs

1 d

Sexual problems and marital difficulties occur in approximately 12% of psychiatric clinic attendees. Swan M, Wilson LJ. Sexual and marital problems in a psychiatric out-patient population. *B J Psychiatry*. 1979; **135**: 310–14.

2 c

A meta-analysis found a twofold increased risk of schizophrenia following cannabis use.
Arseneault L, Cannon M, Witton J *et al*. Causal association between cannabis and psychosis: examination of the evidence. *Br J Psychiatry*. 2004; **184**: 110–17.

3 d

4 b

The point prevalence of depressive symptoms is 10–30% (Puri, Hall, p. 391).

5 c

6 b

(Puri, Hall, p. 294.)

7 c

It was shown in the British Psychiatric Morbidity Survey that 1% of 16–65-year-olds will have suicidal ideation every week.

8 c

9 e

The AESOP study showed that all psychoses were three times as common in black and ethnic minority groups in the UK compared to the white British population (Kirkbride J, Fearon P, Morgan C *et al.* Heterogeneity in incidence rates of schizophrenia and other psychotic syndromes: findings from the 3-Center ÆSOP Study. *Arch Gen Psychiatry.* 2006; **63**: 250–8.).

10 c

The prevalence of insomnia is particularly high in the elderly (Puri, Hall, p. 459).

11 d

The National Confidential Inquiry shows that 5% of perpetrators of homicide have schizophrenia. This is higher than would be expected by chance.

12 c

(Puri, Hall, p. 345.)

13 a

As described by Munro (Puri, Hall, p. 381).

14 e

Males have a higher rate of relapse.

15 c

Cross-cultural studies have shown widely differing rates.

16 d

Dependent personality disorder is the most frequently reported (Puri, Hall, p. 475).

17 d

This has been shown via meta-analysis (Anthony JC, Aboraya A. The epidemiology of selected mental disorders in later life. In: Birren JE,

Sloane RB, Cohen GD, editors. *Handbook of Mental Health and Aging.*
Orlando: Academic Press Inc; 1992. pp. 27–73.).

18 b

19 e

The male to female sex ratio for Tourette's syndrome is 2:1 (Puri, Hall,
p. 491).

20 b

Prevalence of premenstrual syndrome increases with increasing parity
(Puri, Hall, pp. 427–8).

21 e

(Puri, Hall, pp. 287–8.)

22 e

23 c

(Gelder, Lopez-Ibor and Andreasen, p. 593.)

24 b

Female gender is associated with a higher rate of depression.

25 b

Refugees have a high rate of psychiatric morbidity.

26 d

27 c

(Puri, Hall, p. 285.)

28 b

29 e

(Puri, Hall, p. 352.)

30 d

(Puri, Hall, pp. 407–13.)

31 d

32 a

This has been shown by Salib and Cortina-Borja (Salib E, Cortina-Borja M. Effect of month of birth on the risk of suicide. *Br J Psychiatry*. 2006; **188**: 416–22).

33 d

(Puri, Hall, p. 414.)

34 a

35 e

36 c

EMIs

1 1   i

   2   e

   3   d

   4   c

2 1   d, e, i

   2   b, c, j

7

Research and statistics

Questions

MCQs

1 Which of the following is a test for parametric data?

  a *t*-test

  b Wilcoxon

  c Chi-squared test

  d Spearman's rank

  e Mann-Whitney U-test

2 Which of the following is not an advantage of a case-control study?

  a Cheap and quick

  b Can be used to study rare diseases

  c Can investigate a variety of exposures for a single disease

  d Can be used if there is a long time lag between exposure and outcome

  e Can be used to study rare exposures

3 For the values 1, 4, 1, 3, 1, which of the following is false?

  a The mode is 1.

  b The mean is 2.

  c The mean is higher than the mode.

  d The median is 3.

  e The range is 3.

4 Which of the following statements about statistics is false?

   a The variance is a measure of central tendency.

   b The power of a test is the probability that the null hypothesis will be correctly rejected.

   c Parametric tests can be applied as long as one of the variables is measured on an interval or ratio scale.

   d A type II error is that of incorrectly rejecting the alternative hypothesis.

   e A one-tailed test is used if differences are hypothesised to occur in only one direction.

5 Which of the following statements concerning validity is correct?

   a Face validity is the extent to which all aspects of the subject matter are assessed.

   b Convergent validity is a form of criterion validity.

   c Concurrent validity is the extent to which the criterion validity of a measure is retained when applied to a new set of subjects.

   d Cross-validity is the comparison of simultaneous measures involving reference to an external measure.

   e Predictive validity is the ability to predict outcome as measured now and in the future or on another scale.

6 Which of the following is true regarding correlation?

   a It examines the extent to which two variables are causally related.

   b Spearman's rank correlation coefficient can only be applied to normally distributed variables.

   c It is usually expressed along a scale of 0 to 1.

   d It can be assessed using regression analysis.

   e Pearson's product-moment correlation coefficient has the same units as the data.

7 Which of the following statements about statistics is false?

   a The Wilcoxon rank sum test is a non-parametric test.

b The median is greater than the mode in a positively skewed sample.

c The chi-square test cannot be used for the analysis of qualitative data.

d In a normal distribution, 95% of the sample lies within two standard deviations of the mean.

e The standard deviation of the sample distribution is known as the standard error.

A hypothetical study compares diagnoses of depression made by a screening tool used in primary care with those made by psychiatrists using a semi-structured interview that is considered to be a gold standard for the diagnosis of depression. The results are shown in the table below, which should be used to answer questions 8–12.

Primary care screening tool	Semi-structured interview		
	Depression diagnosed	No depression diagnosed	Total
Depression diagnosed	25	20	45
No depression diagnosed	15	60	75
Total	40	80	120

8 The sensitivity of the primary care tool is:

a 55%

b 62.5%

c 75%

d 80%

e 90%

9 The specificity of the primary care tool is:

   a 55%

   b 62.5%

   c 75%

   d 80%

   e 90%

10 The positive predictive value of the primary care tool is:

   a 55%

   b 62.5%

   c 75%

   d 80%

   e 90%

11 The negative predictive value of the tool is:

   a 55%

   b 62.5%

   c 75%

   d 80%

   e 90%

12 The likelihood ratio of a positive test is:

   a 0.5

   b 2.75

   c 0.80

   d 2.5

   e 0.625

13 Bias can:

   a Be introduced only by researchers

   b Occur only at certain stages of the research process

   c Lead to results that differ systematically from the truth

   d Be completely avoided

   e Occur only in certain types of studies

14 Which of these is not a potential cause of a meta-analysis being unreliable?

a Weighting of studies

b Location bias

c Inclusion bias

d Heterogeneity of studies

e Publication bias

15 Which of the following potential explanations of an association is not possible in a prospective cohort study?

a Bias

b Causality

c Random effect

d Confounding

e Reverse causality

16 The standard deviation:

a Can be used for data with a Gaussian distribution

b Is the same as the standard error in the general population

c Equals the variance squared

d Is the numerator in the calculation of parametric effect sizes

e Is the spread of all the observations around the median

A randomized control trial is conducted to assess the use of a new atypical antipsychotic for use in psychosis. It is compared to placebo. A comparison is made between recovery rates in the two groups. This is shown in the table below, which should be used to answer questions 17 and 18.

Group	Recovery	No recovery	Total
New antipsychotic	70	30	100
Placebo	40	55	95

17 The absolute risk reduction (ARR) is:

   a 0.05

   b 0.28

   c 0.66

   d 1.66

   e 3.57

18 The number needed to treat (NNT) is:

   a 1

   b 2

   c 4

   d 9

   e 20

19 The ideal number needed to treat is:

   a 1

   b 2

   c 5

   d 10

   e 20

20 Which of the following is true regarding reliability and testing?

   a Test-retest reliability signifies the internal consistency of a measure or test.

   b Split-half reliability signifies the stability of a test or measure.

   c Sensitivity is the degree to which a test or measure is able to distinguish and exclude those without the disease.

   d Positive predictive value is the proportion correctly described by a test as not having the disease.

   e Inter-rater reliability is the degree of agreement between different raters assessing the same parameters within the same time-frame.

21 Which of the following statements about statistics is true?

   a The Mann-Whitney test is a parametric test.

b The *t*-test is used with qualitative data.

c The Wilcoxon rank sum test involves ranking data from the smallest value to the largest.

d Spearman's rank correlation coefficient is denoted by r.

e In applying the chi-square test, if the expected cell frequencies are small then the F ratio can be used instead.

22 Statistical power is not dependent on:

a Sample size

b Temporality

c Prevalence of the exposure

d Significance level

e Strength of the expected association

23 Which of the following is not an advantage of a randomised control trial?

a It avoids recall bias.

b It precludes selection bias.

c The effects of confounders are eliminated by equal distribution.

d It can evaluate distant and multiple exposures.

e It allows for meta-analysis.

24 Sensitivity is:

a The proportion of people with the disorder who have a positive test

b The probability of a positive test coming from someone with a disorder compared to someone without the disorder

c The proportion of people with a positive test who actually have the disorder

d The proportion of people with a negative test who do not have the disorder

e The proportion of people without the disorder who have a negative test

25 A hypothetical cohort study follows all the babies born in one year in one inner-city hospital until the age of 25 years. Cannabis use is established by interviewing the patients, and hospital records are used to establish any cases of schizophrenia. The results are shown in the table below.

	Schizophrenia	No schizophrenia
Cannabis use	24	3600
No cannabis use	6	4400

The relative risk (RR) of schizophrenia in the cannabis users is:
a 0.005
b 0.21
c 0.33
d 2.94
e 4.79

26 Which of the following statements about confidence intervals is false?
a It is the range within which the true measure actually lies.
b They give the same information as p values.
c They are a measure of dispersion of data.
d They give the precision of a measure.
e A narrow confidence interval allows more confidence in the results.

27 A case-control study investigated the rate of parental divorce on subsequent development of anxiety disorder (see table below). What is the correct odds ratio (OR)?

	Anxiety disorder	No anxiety disorder
Parental divorce	55	21
No parental divorce	105	227

a 0.4

b 0.52

c 2.25

d 5.78

e 7.62

28 Which of the following statements about survival analysis is false?

a It is useful when the outcome is time until an event.

b Data can be analysed with the log rank test.

c It assumes that dropouts have a different prognosis to those remaining in the study.

d A Kaplan-Meier curve can be used to illustrate the data.

e Data can be analysed with Cox's proportional hazards.

29 Which of the following does not minimise the effect of confounding?

a Blinding

b Restricting the study population

c Matching

d Stratification

e Multivariate analysis

30 Which of the following is false regarding the Mann-Whitney U-test?

a It is a non-parametric version of *t*-test.

b It can be used for ordinal, interval or ratio variables.

c It can be used to compare the means of two independent groups.

d It is based on rank values.

e Results should be presented as a median with a description of the skew (e.g. box plot).

31 Which of the following is not a disadvantage of a cohort study?

    a It takes a long period of time.

    b It is not suitable for rare exposures.

    c Loss to follow-up may lead to selection bias.

    d Exposure status may change in the unexposed group.

    e Non-participation of those eligible may limit generalisability.

32 Specificity is:

    a The proportion of people with the disorder who have a positive test

    b The probability of a positive test coming from someone with a disorder compared to someone without the disorder

    c The proportion of people with a positive test who actually have the disorder

    d The proportion of people with a negative test who do not have the disorder

    e The proportion of people without the disorder who have a negative test

33 Which of the following is false regarding regression?

    a Multiple regression can evaluate the role of confounders.

    b In the equation $y = a + bx$, b is the regression coefficient.

    c Logistic regression can be used when the dependent variable is binary.

    d Regression is the prediction of an independent variable based on its relationship with another, dependent variable.

    e Multiple regression can be used when the dependent variable is continuous.

34 Which one of these does not increase the likelihood that the observed association is true?

a Temporality

b Dose-response relationship

c Biological plausibility

d Consistency

e Relative risk of 1.5

35 Which of these statements about confounders is false?

a Age and sex are common confounders.

b They are on the causal pathway between exposure and the disease.

c They are best identified at the design stage of a study.

d They can be controlled for statistically.

e They are associated with both the exposure and the disease.

36 Which of the following is a test for non-parametric data?

a Independent *t*-test

b Analysis of variance

c Chi-squared test

d Multiple linear regression

e Paired *t*-test

37 Which method can be used to evaluate the possibility of publication bias in a meta-analysis?

a Funnel plot

b F statistic

c Confidence interval of the summary effect size

d Log rank test

e P value of the summary effect size

EMIs

1 Statistical tests:

a Paired *t*-test

b Chi-squared test

c Multiple regression

d McNemar test

e ANOVA

f Independent *t*-test

g Logistic regression

h Mann–Whitney U-test

i Pearson's product moment correlation

j Bonferroni correction

k Kruskal-Wallis test

l Spearman rank correlation

A group of researchers conducted a randomised control trial of venlafaxine versus mirtazapine in a group of depressed patients using the Hamilton Rating Scale for Depression. Choose the most appropriate test for each of the following analyses they want to conduct.

1 They want to know if age and gender have any effect on treatment.

2 They want to find out if there are any age differences between the venlafaxine and mirtazapine groups.

3 They want to find out if there are any gender differences between the venlafaxine and the mirtazapine groups. (2 answers)

2 Study designs:

   a Case-control study

   b Double-blind randomised control trial

   c Cohort study

   d Ecological study

   e Systematic review

   f Cross-sectional survey

   g Single-blind randomised control trial

   h Meta-analysis

   i Qualitative study

What would be the ideal study design to answer the following questions?

   1 You want to compare with lithium the effectiveness of a newly released mood stabiliser.

   2 You wish to know more about the reasons why patients stop taking their medication.

   3 Conflicting existing data exists about the impact of cannabis use on the risk of schizophrenia. You want to know what the overall effect is.

   4 You would like to know whether babies born in urban areas have a greater risk of developing ADHD than those born in rural areas.

3 Biases:

   a Publication bias

   b Recall bias

   c Sampling bias

   d Observer bias

   e Information bias

   f Responder bias

   g Measurement bias

Match the situations below with the types of bias listed above.

  1 A study into the effectiveness of an antipsychotic for schizo-phrenia excludes all patients with any type of co-morbidity.

  2 A study asks mothers of young people with schizophrenia whether they experienced obstetric complications.

  3 A study into the effectiveness of cognitive-behavioural therapy compares only hospital notes.

4 Study designs:
  a Case-control study
  b Double-blind randomised control trial
  c Cohort study
  d Ecological study
  e Systematic review
  f Cross-sectional study
  g Single-blind randomised control trial
  h Meta-analysis
  i Qualitative study

Which type of studies are described below?

  1 Trainee psychiatrists were invited to a focus group to elicit their views on the new examination system.

  2 All babies born in a town in one year were followed up until their eighteenth birthday.

  3 A survey was sent to all patients who were currently under the care of a community mental health team, which included demographic information such as gender and ethnicity.

  4 Patients attending a CMHT with OCD were randomly assigned to receive either CBT or an SSRI. The psychiatrist assessing outcome was not aware of what treatment the patient had received.

Answers

MCQs

1 a

2 e

Rare exposures are difficult to investigate using case-control studies.

3 d

The median is 1. It is the middle value when the numbers are ranked in order.

4 a

Variance is a measure of dispersion.

5 e

6 d

7 c

The chi-square test is a non-parametric test.

8 b

Sensitivity = 25/40 = 0.625 = 62.5%

9 c

Specificity = 60/80 = 0.75 = 75%

10 a

Positive predictive value = 25/45 = 0.55 = 55%

11 d

Negative predictive value = 60/75 = 0.8 = 80%

12 d

Likelihood ratio of a positive test = sensitivity/1-specificity.

13 c

Bias can be defined as any process at any stage of the process that tends to produce results that differ systematically from the truth. There are several types of bias that can be introduced by the researchers or the subjects themselves (Lawrie, McIntosh, Rao, p. 43).

14 a

Weighting of the results of studies in a meta-analysis according to size and quality allows larger, higher-quality studies to have relatively more influence on the summary effect size (Lawrie, McIntosh, Rao, p. 40).

15 e

16 a

Gaussian is another term for normal distribution (Lawrie, McIntosh, Rao, pp. 59–60).

17 b

ARR = experimental event rate (EER) – control event rate (CER) = 0.7 – 0.42 = 0.28

18 c

NNT = 1/ARR = 1/0.28 = 3.6

19 a

This would mean that every patient treated has a favourable outcome.

20 e

21 c

22 b

23 d

Evaluating distant and multiple exposures is an advantage of a case-control design.

24 a

25 e

Relative risk (RR) = 24/3600 divided by 6/4400 = 0.0067/0.0014 = 4.79

26 b

They give all the information of a p value plus the precision of any estimate (Lawrie, McIntosh, Rao, p. 62).

27 d

OR = 55/105 divided by 21/227 = 0.52/0.09 = 5.78

28 c

Survival analysis assumes that dropouts have the same prognosis as those remaining in the study (Johnstone, Cunningham-Owens and Lawrie, p. 189).

29 a

30 c

It is used to compare the medians, not means (Johnstone, Cunningham-Owens and Lawrie, p. 194).

31 b

A cohort study is good for rare exposures but not suitable for rare outcomes.

32 e

33 d

Regression is the prediction of a dependent variable based on its relationship with another, independent, variable (Lawrie, McIntosh, Rao, p. 257).

34 e

A relative risk of 1.5 should be treated with caution; a relative risk of 2 or above is more likely to indicate causality.

35 b

A confounder is a variable associated with both exposure and outcome that does not lie on the causal pathway (Lawrie, McIntosh, Rao, p. 252).

36 c

37 a

EMIs

1 1 g

     2 f

     3 b, d

2 1 b

     2 i

     3 h

     4 c

3   1   c

     2   b

     3   e

4   1   i

     2   c

     3   f

     4   g

Index

Key: (Q) = question, (A) = answer

£21·95